Imagineering
for Health

Serge King

IMAGINEERING FOR HEALTH

*This publication made possible with
the assistance of the Kern Foundation*

The Theosophical Publishing House
Wheaton, Ill. U.S.A.
Madras, India/London, England

Fourth Quest printing 1987

Library of Congress Catalog Number: 80-53949
ISBN: 0-8356-0546-9

Printed in the United States of America

PART III — TECHNIQUES

Introduction

This is a book about creating a state of health in yourself, using your own spiritual, mental, and emotional resources. "Imagineering" is the term I use for doing that, because it implies the process of building something with your mind. There are virtually no limits to what you can do with Imagineering, but the focus here will be on healing.

What you'll be reading is a kind of distillation of nearly thirty years of research into the nature of the human mind and emotions. As a student of metaphysics, a paraphysicist, an amateur anthropologist, a social engineer, a management consultant, a pastoral counselor, and a psychologist I've had some unique opportunities to study the positive and negative effects of human thinking. During that time I've become absolutely convinced that we create our own experience, that we are victims only of ourselves, and that we have the power to remake our experience in almost any fashion we choose.

The most outstanding example of that power lies in our own state of health. While spending seven years in Africa and associating off and on with various "medicine men" I witnessed many instances of what most Americans might call miraculous healings. I've seen the same kind of "miracles" in the company of spiritual and psychic healers in this country, and, using what I learned, I've achieved some pretty remarkable things myself. In addition, while studying to become a psychologist, I've grown to realize more and more that healing is not a special ability reserved for a few highly trained experts or "unusual" people, but a natural, creative skill that every human being possesses. We create our illness as we create our health, and in the final analysis no one can cure us but ourselves. What keeps everyone from realizing that is simply their beliefs about what healing and illness are.

And so I begin my book by talking about ideas and beliefs and how they determine what we experience. Then I acquaint you with some powers and characteristics of your mind that you may not yet fully appreciate. In Part II of the book I discuss many of the ways in which we create illness, and in Part III I give you a variety of ways to begin creating health.

It's a book full of unorthodox ideas, I freely admit. Some of them might even make orthodox health practitioners hot under the collar. But it's an honest book. Every idea has been successfully used by someone. My purpose is to put the power of healing back where it belongs—with YOU. I'm not advocating the total overthrow of our present health system by any means because it can and does do an immense amount of good work. But I wouldn't mind a little revolution to get things back into proper perspective. This book is about you and for you. Read it. Use it. Get healthy.

CHAPTER ONE

The World Is What You Think It Is

Ideas rule the world. There are two kinds of ideas that rule the world, however—facts and opinions. And each one produces different kinds of effects.

A fact, the way I define it, is something that affects every human being on earth, regardless of race, creed, culture or location. Actually, there are relatively few facts. Life is a fact. So are birth, death, gravity, electromagnetism, the earth, the sun, air, heat, cold, etc. Facts are things which *are*. They and the effects they produce affect everyone. And for all practical purposes they can't be changed. You can eliminate facts (like humans eliminated the dodo bird) and you can manipulate them (to make refrigerators and electric lights) but you can't change the facts themselves.

To make this as clear as possible, I will explain that I include material things, as well as ideas, as facts. For if you accept the dodo bird, the dinosaur, and the passenger pigeon as facts, then it is obvious that those "facts" have ceased to exist. One cannot change the fact of existence of the dodo or the passenger pigeon somewhere in time, but by killing off all of them one can eliminate that fact as part of present reality. If a fact is *what is*, then a dodo bird is not

1

a fact because it isn't. What is, in the case of the poor dodo, is the record of the bird. The record is fact, the bird is not. This is why I say that facts can be eliminated and manipulated, but not changed.

The largest category of ideas that affect our lives consists of opinions, which in this book I am equating with beliefs. Opinions are ideas *about* facts, and they only affect some of the people some of the time. Nevertheless, they are very potent, because it is your opinions about life that determine how you feel, what you do, how you relate to other people and all the rest of your personal experience. Opinions differ markedly from facts in that they can be changed. And as opinions change, so do your experiences of facts.

What gets many people into trouble is that they tend to confuse opinions with facts. In other words, they treat their opinions as facts of life, rather than of ideas about facts. Typical opinions that some people call facts are:

"Life is a struggle."
"Success is due to luck."
"Whatever happens is due to fate."
"I am powerless against the forces around me."
"I am incompetent and unworthy."
"The world is a loving and exciting place."
"I can do anything I set my mind on."
"Experience is predictable (or unpredictable)."

To clarify what I'm saying, let me extract the facts from the above opinions:

"Life is."
"Success is."
"Whatever happens is."
"I am."
"The world is."
"I can do."
"Experience is."

Those are the facts. *Anything added to them is an opinion.* As you can see, opinions may be either positive or negative. What matters, though, is that whichever they are, they will govern what you experience. An opinion about life is something like a special set of filtered glasses through which you look out on the world. They are so special that they only allow you to see certain things in a certain way.

With your filtered opinion glasses you block out of your awareness anything which can't pass through the filter, so life appears to conform to your pre-set opinion. Instead of reacting freely to what is, you react to what your opinions tell you. If this works for you—if it makes you healthier, happier, stronger, more successful, etc., then that's great. As you examine yourself and the people around you, though, you may find that all too often your glasses—your opinions—aren't working for you. Don't despair. Opinions are not facts. You chose (at some level) the ones you have, and you don't have to keep them if you don't want to.

The Source of Your Opinions

You may be wondering about now, "If my beliefs about life are just opinions, how did I get them in the first place?" Okay, I'll tell you.

From the moment you came out of the womb, you began experiencing life in full, and you began trying to understand what was going on around you. As a baby you aren't just a hunk of squirming flesh. You are much more aware and responsive to your environment than most people think. Recently I read an article saying that newborn infants only sixty seconds old were able to make imitations and responses to the facial gestures of an adult. Along with responding you are making your first attempts to interpret your experience, too. As you grow you have to try and make some sense out of this new world, and so you make choices or decisions about what your experience means. Once you have made a tentative decision, you automatically look around for confirmation that your decision makes sense, that it is "correct."

Your parents are very helpful in this regard. You watch their responses to various events, hear their words, listen to their telepathy, and use that data for making and confirming your decisions. Some of what they do, say and think you accept, and some of it you reject. One of the current psychological projects has to do with the study of children who are called "invulnerables." These are simply children who grow up in households with chaotic, schizophrenic, neurotic and/or psychopathic parents and siblings, and who don't seem to be affected by the ideas and behavior of the rest of the family. They aren't genetically or otherwise superior to children who do succumb. They have just made different decisions about life and about themselves. You see, you aren't a helpless, blank slate on which all your parents' opinions are written. You choose all along the way. When you get a little older, you observe and listen to relatives, playmates and authoritative adults, and continue to make decisions. The simple fact that children from the same family can grow up with such different personalities shows that their decisions were individually made.

Once you have decided that a particular choice of how to interpret an experience is correct, you have given birth to an opinion. From them on you will tend to channel all similar experiences through the same opinion, paying attention only to those parts of the experience that confirm your choice and ignoring the rest. Most of the big decisions you make about life occur in childhood, and they act as guidelines right through adulthood unless you change them.

Let's look at two young children who have brought a bucket of water and some dirt into the house and are making mud pies on the dining room table. Their mother comes in and is aghast. She shouts and screams, tells them how bad they are, and gives them a sound spanking. That is the raw experience. But one of them chooses to focus on the idea that he is bad, that he has hurt mother somehow, and that he must be very dumb not to have figured out what he was doing was wrong. This confirms earlier tentative decisions that the world is unpredictable and he is pretty incapable of dealing with it. The second child chooses to focus on the idea that parents don't like dirt, that he is likely to get a spanking if he does things they don't like, and that there are plenty of other places to make mud pies. This confirms earlier tentative decisions that the world is unpredictable and that he is capable of dealing with it. The same raw experience processed through two different sets of filters produces two completely individual sets of guidelines.

You are the source of your experience because your decisions about life color your thoughts, your imagination, your emotions, and your actions. And all these serve like a magnet for associated events, circumstances, and people, attracting you to them and them to you. There's an awful lot of life out there in the world. The part of it that you experience is a result of your opinions about it.

Your Life Reflects Your Opinions

It is one thing to understand with your intellect that you are the source of your experience. It is quite another thing to take a close look at your life and say, "Whoops! Look at what I did!" This is a pretty hard idea to accept, especially in a society which tends to promote the idea that life is something that happens to you. But successful people are those who do have the willingness to accept that they happen to life, not the other way around.

Before you can begin to choose better opinions, you have to recognize the ones you now have that aren't working. One way is to take a good look at your present experience, and to realize that any of its characteristics, desirable and undesirable, are the effects of your own thinking. The state of your life is a dead giveaway to the state of your beliefs. Boy, I have had a lot of people argue with me on that one! They insisted that their beliefs about life were all pristine pure and positive, while their experience was a shambles. Not until they were able to overcome their fear of really looking into their own minds were we able to make any progress in improving their experience. There is no way to get around it: If you are living in poverty, you are holding opinions, that keep you from getting money; if you have poor health, you are holding opinions that are keeping you from becoming well; if you can't get along with people, you are holding opinions that keep you from doing so. What is in your life reflects what is in your mind.

Your life is a mirror for your beliefs about it, but looking at your life merely tells you in which areas of life your beliefs are or are not working for you. It doesn't tell you exactly what the beliefs are. That requires a little more self-examination, and I'll give you an exercise for that at the end of the book. For the moment I'll show you some examples of what kind of beliefs can produce given experiences.

The following partial outline of a belief system was taken from a person I was training who realized that the money aspect of her life just wasn't working. By a process of self-questioning we found that her basic opinion about money was that

MONEY IS TIME

Then, of course, we had to find out her basic opinion about time, which was

TIME IS LIMITED

These two opinions produced the following logical sequence in her biocomputer:

Time is limited,
and Money is Time,
therefore, Money is limited,
therefore, no matter how hard I work or
how much I earn, I will never have enough
Money.

Since we can only act according to our basic opinions about life, this woman was habitually creating conditions through her behavior to make her experience conform to what she believed about money.

To show how different opinions can produce the same effect, here is another example. In this case it was a man who held the following three basic opinions about life:

YOU ALWAYS GET WHAT YOU DESERVE
I AM A GOOD PERSON
MONEY IS BAD

which inevitably led to

I deserve what is good, and therefore, I don't deserve money.

It might be humorous except that it was playing havoc with this man's life. Don't fail to note that the same effect (a lack of money) would again be produced if the second two beliefs were "I am a bad person" and "Money is good." There's more than one way to skin a cat, if I may be permitted to express another popular opinion about life.

All Problems Are Caused By a Conflict of Ideas

Mental, emotional, social, and physical experiences of pain, suffering and lack all have their roots in a conflict of opinions or ideas. Of several types of conflict, one that causes the most trouble is based on "should be" opinions. What I mean by that is an idea that something "should be" different than what it appears to be. Suppose you are a mother with a nice, deep-seated opinion that housework is drudgery. In various and subtle ways you have communicated this idea to your children, who have accepted it avidly. However, you also have an opinion that children should keep their room neat and clean (not that children do it, but that they *should* do it.) What will probably happen is that the children's room will usually look like a disaster area and you will work yourself into a fit of frustration, nagging, and perhaps headaches or stomach upsets because their room isn't kept the way it "should be." Children should be neat, but they aren't, but they should be, but they aren't, but they should be—and so goes your head.

"Should be's" can crop up in any area of life with potentially devastating effects on health and efficiency. What is so bad about them is that they are designed to make you a loser no matter what you do. They generate conflict by the very nature of their suppositions. The use of the word "should" in this sense implies beforehand that it doesn't correspond to what is (aside from the fact that "what is" is still only your idea of what is). So you go on comparing what you are experiencing with what you "should be" experiencing, and end up in constant battle with yourself.

One of the most common "should be" ideas is represented by the cry, "That isn't fair!" Naturally, that implies that whatever isn't fair should be. People who use that statement a lot tend to experience a lot of unhappiness. The general idea that supports it is "Life should be fair." In order to reach the foundation of that one, you have to find out what is meant by "fair." What you'll find, if you dig deep, is that it translates into "Life should be the way I want it to be." Once that meaning is recognized, you'll have a clearer choice as to whether to continue with such an opinion or change it. Note that there is a big difference between "Life *should* be the way I want it to be" and "Life *can* be the way I want it to be." The first one stifles positive effort, the second encourages it. So watch out for the "should be's" in your life. You'll be a lot happier, more effective, and have a greater sense of confidence and self-worth if you get rid of them.

Another type of conflict occurs when an idea about generalizations runs smack up against an idea about specifics. A sergeant I knew in the Marine Corps came to me one day to unload his troubles. He was a Southerner, and his problem had to do with the fact that we had a racially mixed platoon. *Individually,* he got along with the blacks in our barracks because each one was friendly, hard-working, and supportive of our team effort. When he thought of them and reacted to them as men, he had no problem. But when he thought of them as blacks, all the old feelings he had been brought up with came out and he was in a turmoil. The prejudicial opinions he had learned as a child were still current beliefs, but they didn't hold up at all when he dealt with specific people. The statement that "Some of my best friends are black" is often taken as a cliche for hypocrisy, but maybe it isn't. It could be just an awkward recognition of the conflict between an honest generalized opinion and opinions about specific people. But such conflicts still cause unnecessary fear, separation, and social conflict. You may find such conflicts within yourself between generalizations and specifics dealing with race, religion, politics, culture, education, fame, and fortune. Examine them well. If the generalizations don't make you happier, healthier, more loving and more effective, maybe they aren't worth keeping.

Inner conflicts, with their outer effects, also occur when an old opinion is being challenged by a new one. Our opinions about the world are intimately connected to our sense of security. Strange as it seems, even old opinions that are no longer effective or that are causing us all kinds of trouble still offer a kind of security because we are used to them. When we choose or are "forced by circumstances" to interpret our reality in a new way, we invariably go through a period of insecurity before the new interpretation is established as a habit. The more fundamental the belief which is being challenged, the greater the sense of insecurity. Sometimes it can literally seem as if the world is falling apart. And in such a case it's true; our old world is breaking up because experience follows belief. *But you won't have positive changes in your life unless the desire to alter your circumstances is greater than the comfort of familiar pain.*

The Present Is 'Where It's At'

Now is all there is. Although we live in a time-oriented world, all you can ever experience is the present moment. What we call the past is just a bunch of other present moments, remembered or recorded and experienced as knowledge in this present. And the future is just a bunch of present moments yet to be experienced, but which we can think about in this present.

A large number of people think that the causes for their present difficulties lie in the past. That isn't quite the way it is. It is true that in the past you made certain decisions about life, and that these decisions produced the effects you now experience, but you are experiencing those effects now because your thinking is still operating according to those old decisions. Decisions about life are like seeds with an inner urge to fulfill their own potential. Apples grow from apple seeds, but the seeds don't cause the apples. What causes the apples is the continuing urge toward fulfillment. It doesn't matter whether the decisions have produced happy or unhappy effects, apples, or weeds. The urge toward fulfillment is there and the effects will continue until you uproot the plants you don't want.

Many people also have been given the idea that present difficulties are caused by memories of past incidents that are buried deep in some unconscious part of the self. The image of the psychiatrist who must spend months or years uncovering some traumatic incident from the past that is secretly affecting a patient's behavior is well known to the general public. My approach is quite different in three ways.

First, for all practical purposes the past no longer exists: your *memory* of it does. But your memory exists in the present and very often it doesn't agree with other people's memory about the same experiences. Have you ever talked about old times with a friend or a relative, only to find that their memory of what happened at a particular time is not the same as yours at all? It isn't a question of who is right, but of how each one of you interpreted the experience and modified it to fit your beliefs. You remember what you do because of your present opinions. As your opinions change, so do your memories and your reactions to those memories. In the case of one woman I helped, she was unable at first to recall any happy incidents from her childhood. As far as she was concerned it was a black and bitter period. After a few sessions on changing opinions, however, she suddenly began to recall numerous happy incidents. Those memories weren't buried anywhere. They were available all the time. She just wasn't looking at them. In addition, she began looking at the bitter incidents in a different light and realizing that they weren't so bad after all. Before, she would have sworn on a holy book that her memory of the past was the only true one.

Second, past incidents are relatively unimportant. It is easy to spend years going through and picking apart memories of past incidents that you can blame for current situations, but that is slow, tedious, unnecessary, and often unproductive. It's like picking away the mortar from around individual bricks in a big wall. It's much easier, faster, and more effective to uproot the foundation, because then the whole wall falls down. When a basic opinion about life is changed, then every incident and associated opinion is changed as well. The memory of the incidents remain, but their interpretation—and therefore their effect on you—is totally altered. A woman I worked with had severe learning disabilities which she blamed on having been told as a child that she was mentally retarded. She had gone the shrink route, but all that gave her were some incidents on which to hang her blame. The only thing

I did was to show her that she was still holding onto the opinion that she couldn't learn difficult subjects. With encouragement, in a comparatively short time she was able to change that opinion, and now she is successfully taking courses in astronomy, physics, and biochemistry. By the way, I am not knocking psychiatrists. I'm just saying that some of their methods are not very effective.

Third, I hold that all your opinions are consciously available at any moment. They aren't locked away in some dark dungeon of your subconscious where they are jealously guarded against your perception. You know, consciously, exactly what they are. It's just that sometimes you forget they are there, or you don't want to look at them. You have an awful lot of information in your conscious mind that you take for granted and don't pay any attention to. For instance, there is Afghanistan. Now, I don't know what your opinion of Afghanistan is, but you know, and you can bring it into awareness if you want to. Of course, if I hadn't mentioned Afghanistan you might not have thought about it for weeks, but the information is there, available. And so is the information about all your other, more pertinent opinions. The main reason some of them may be hard to bring to your immediate attention is that there are probably some strong "should not" opinions interfering. Suppose you have an opinion to the effect that "My mother is a real bitch." You may also have another opinion that says "I shouldn't feel that way about my mother." If the second one is stronger it can keep you from looking at the first, and you may do a good job of convincing yourself that you don't understand why you can't get along with her. The point is that just because you don't want to look at particular opinions, that doesn't mean you don't know you have them. Besides, their effects are all around you.

As for the future, there is nothing set about it whatsoever. It grows out of your present thoughts, including the habitual ones you don't pay much attention to. You are planting the seeds for your future right now. Because you have the power to change your thoughts, however, the future is a series of probabilities instead of a fixed destiny. You are by no means a victim of the past, nor of the present either. Past habits in thought and behavior do not determine your future unless you let them, and you don't have to let them. As the saying goes, you reap what you sow. Your thoughts are the seeds, your emotions the fertilizer, and planting time is now.

Your Only Limitations Are The Ones You Agree To

As a human being, you really don't have many limitations. Sitting here racking my brains, I find it very hard to come up with any limitations that haven't been overcome by someone somewhere at some time. And since we all come from the same stock, what is possible for one human is potentially possible for any other human.

Youth is not a limitation. There have been child prodigies in almost every field of endeavor, and recent studies have shown that the IQ's of apparently dumb children can be dramatically raised simply by giving them a teacher who believes they are smarter than they have previously shown themselves to be; during the American Revolution we had captains of ships who were sixteen and nineteen years old; more recently we have many examples of people under twenty-five, including teenagers, who have become successful businessmen, some of them millionaires; and we are seeing more and more youngsters in their early teens becoming Olympic stars.

Old age is not a limitation. There are seniors in their eighties successfully starting new careers; some seniors are physically vital enough to perform amazing feats of strength and endurance in such sports as swimming, weight-lifting and running; and many seniors are successfully sharing their wisdom and expertise in various areas of social development, including some I knew as Peace Corps volunteers in Africa.

The state of one's body is not a limitation. People with severe physical disabilities have turned themselves into star athletes; others have learned to use their minds to make a success in business or politics or education (my excellent teacher of Shakespeare in college was blind); missing limbs can be replaced by prostheses; and people who are ordinarily weak have, under stress, lifted vehicles to free trapped victims of accidents.

Poverty is not a limitation. Andrew Carnegie started out as a pauper, and so did a host of others mentioned frequently in self-help books.

Being part of an ethnic minority is not a limitation. Although there are still civil rights and opportunities yet to be won, blacks, chicanos, and others have shown that they can be successful in every field that I know of.

Being a woman is not a limitation. Again, there are still prejudices to be overcome and rights to be won for women as a whole, but women too have shown their ability to succeed in any area.

Being an ex-convict is not a limitation. In spite of social prejudice, ex-convicts have gone on to become lawyers, famous writers, and successful businessmen.

I have given these few examples to emphasize the fact that whatever you think your limitations may be, they are only limitations because you think they are. And as long as you continue to think of them as preventing you from doing what you desire to accomplish, they will do just that. If you want to get out of the trap, don't think of them as limitations at all, but as conditions or factors that you have to take into account in your approach to successful living. What one person can do, you can do. Maybe you aren't interested in doing it to the same extent, but you can do it to the degree that pleases you. Seen as conditions to deal with, limitations no longer are barriers on your path of life, but the state of the trail itself. Rocky, slippery, twisting, or steep, the condition of your path only determines what you have to do to get to the end; it doesn't stop you from getting there. You do that to yourself by sitting down and complaining about the way the path looks instead of moving on. And you have the potential for smoothing it out.

Change Your Opinions and Choose Your Experience

That's what this chapter is all about—to get you to realize that you are the master of your personal destiny. Experience follows belief, and you have the power to change whatever beliefs or opinions that are ineffective in giving you the experience you want.

Now, I am not promising instant results. Sometimes that does happen, but more often it doesn't. The reason has to do with what I call "experiential momentum." That's a fancy phrase for the fact that the experiences we have created from our thoughts tend to keep going for awhile even after we have changed our thinking. Another way of saying it is that we often have to live with the fruits of our past opinions for a certain time. How long they last depends on how long we've had them, how much emotion was involved with them, how completely we've changed our opinions, and how much emotion or desire we put into the new ones. I want you to know this so that you'll beware of discouragement before you achieve results. Changing your opinions does change your experience, but in many cases you'll need patience and persistence to carry it through. Believe me, the rewards are worth it. Successful living is a skill, and like any skill it takes practice to become an expert.

CHAPTER TWO

ThE Tool of ImaqiNATioN

Of all the mental tools used in Imagineering, the most important is imagination itself. The others are important too, but there is no question that this is number one. Imagination is so important because it governs most of the ways you feel and behave. Almost everything you have learned or experienced was preceded by imagination in some form or another. Even as a baby, though you may not remember it, you learned to crawl, walk, and run by first imagining yourself doing it and then following through.

Spontaneous and Willed Imagination

If you have become used to taking your mental activity for granted, you may be surprised to know that you have several kinds of imagination. Two of these kinds are spontaneous imagination and willed imagination. They are different because they originate from different parts or aspects of your mind, which I'll detail in another chapter. For now let's just call them the subconscious and the conscious.

Spontaneous imagination is produced by your subconscious and is formed from memory and telepathic input. Its main characteristic is that it seems to arise of its own accord, or at least the details of the content do. You can consciously decide to recall a memory, but the content of the memory is a subconscious production. You can even consciously decide to be aware of telepathic input, but the input itself is spontaneously offered by the subconscious. When I speak of telepathic input I should mention that I am referring not only to mental communication with other people, but with other parts of yourself as well, including your body. At any rate, spontaneous imagination is largely governed by your existing opinions about yourself and about life, and by your resulting habits of thought. It can be creative, but it is the kind of creativity that mixes elements already on hand. It can create new combinations, but not new concepts.

Willed imagination means just that. It is imagination constructed by a conscious act of will. Note that this is not the same as willing a memory to appear or willing yourself to be aware of telepathic data. What is involved here is willing the content of your imagination, that is, consciously deciding just what the content is going to be. The difference between spontaneous and willed imagination is like the difference between recalling a memory and constructing a daydream of some delightful experience that has never happened and is highly improbable. It is through willed imagination that we develop new concepts and attract new experiences. One of the things that makes humans different from animals is that we can imagine what isn't. Of course, this can be either a burden or an adventure, depending on the content.

In most cases of imagination using the will there is some degree of spontaneous imagination present which acts to "fill in the details" of the imagery. And "pure" spontaneous imagination can be modified or manipulated by adding willed imagination. All of this will serve very practical purposes, as you will see in other parts of this book. Below is an experiment you can perform to demonstrate spontaneous and willed imagination.

Experiment: Imagine a scene of a small village. It has one main street and a building taller than the rest at the end of the street. Do this now before you read any further. Take thirty seconds to a minute to get the scene clear in your mind.

Okay, what kind of scene was it? Were the buildings of thatch, adobe, wood or what? Was the street paved or dirt? Were there any people? What kind of building was at the end of the street? Was the village in India, South America, Europe or elsewhere? Was it a memory of a real village you once visited or saw a picture of, or was it apparently new? This experiment is meant to show you that all the detailed content of the image is produced by your subconscious spontaneous imagination, even if it was an actual memory. In all probability, the village sprang quickly to mind, "full-grown" as it were. You most likely didn't have to consciously insert any of the elements, which proves its spontaneity. Now, however, I would like you to use your conscious will and place yourself and some friend walking down the street of the village and looking at the sights. If you actually did walk down such a street with a friend once, then imagine a different friend with you this time and do different things. Spend a few moments on this.

What you just did was to impose willed imagination into a scene of spontaneous imagination. You may have done something like this before many times in daydreams, but I want you to be aware of it *as a technique* because it will come in very handy as you practice creating your own reality on a conscious level.

Picture and Mime Imagination

Experiment: In your mind, imagine a package about six inches square all tied up with a red ribbon. Imagine yourself opening the package and finding a bracelet inside lying on some cotton. Then imagine putting it on your wrist (if you're a man you can make it a heavy masculine bracelet if you want). Okay, stop. Now imagine the same kind of package sitting in your real, physical lap, as if the package were a three-dimensional reality. Imagine your real hands opening it up in front of you, taking out the bracelet and putting it on your real wrist. Now stop. Can you tell the difference?

If you are like most people, the first image was like a picture projected on a movie screen and you probably saw yourself as another person opening the package and taking out the bracelet. But the second image was probably more realistic and the experience more vivid. That's because it was imagined as a part of your immediate physical environment. It was quite different from the first in terms of the quality of the experience. This kind of imagination also has a greater effect on you physiologically. If I had asked you to imagine a spider inside the package of the first image you probably could have done so without too much reaction. But with the second kind of imagination, it is very likely that your adrenal glands would have shot a bit of juice into your system in spite of yourself.

The point is that here are two more different types of imagination that you have, each with its own characteristics and uses. Your body has a greater response to the second type. This same kind of imagination was at work if you were ever alone in the dark and imagined that someone or something "out there" was ready to pounce on you. Since it resembles the kind of imagination conjured up by a mime during a stage performance (you know, like when someone with their face painted white pretends to be walking down stairs so well that you can almost see the staircase), let's call it "mime imagination." The first kind we'll call "picture imagination."

Picture imagination is good for memory recall, creative play (that some call daydreams), developing new ideas, planning projects, and meditation of various kinds. It makes a great tool for those things.

Mime imagination, on the other hand, is better for actually making improvements in your personality and skills, in your relationships and in your environment, as well as in your health. Many athletes use mime imagination to prepare their minds and "pretrain" their bodies for upcoming events. Good actors use it to create believable characters, and some enlightened businessmen and politicians use it to prepare for meetings and speaking engagements. I once helped two young people on their way to becoming champion skaters by training them in the use of mime imagination. Not only did I help prepare their minds and pretrain their bodies to skate perfectly, but I think I helped them even more by taking them right through the whole process of winning. The training gave them the confidence and positive expectation that sent them on their way to the top.

Multi-sensory Imagination

Generally, when people first hear the word imagination they think of visual images. However, the complete tool of imagination also includes the imagined senses of taste, touch, smell, and hearing.

Experiment: Imagine that you are looking at a rosebush just after a light rain. Right on top is a large rose with its petals fully open. Imagine that you reach out gently to grasp the stem and feel the slight prick of the thorns. Bring the rose to your nose and take a deep smell of its perfume. Imagine there are drops of dew on the petals. Lick some of them off with your tongue and taste the sweet freshness of the water. Now let go of the rose and imagine that a bee comes to land upon it and you can hear the buzzing of its wings.

As you can tell, the above experiment is designed to let you bring all your senses into the imagined scene. When you use imagination in a multisensory way like this it has a much more powerful impact on you, and your thoughts, feelings, and behavior in particular. This is because your subconscious doesn't know the difference between a "real" and an imagined experience. It will respond on a muscular, glandular, cellular, and memory level as much to one as to the other, especially when more than one sense is involved. That might sound hard to believe at first, but the next experiment might help to convince you.

Experiment: Imagine yourself in a spacecraft, circling the earth. You are looking down through a porthole and you can see the continents and oceans below, with cloud formations of various kinds covering parts of them. You can see areas of brown and green, and over the blue ocean you can see a swirling ring of clouds that looks like a hurricane forming. Now be aware of the thick glass of the porthole and touch it with your finger. You are also aware of the cushions of your seat, the spacesuit you are wearing, and the metallic feel of the controls by your hands. There is a slight ozone smell in the air of the spaceship and you can hear instruments whirring and clicking. You also feel the excitement of being on such an adventure so far above the earth. Spend a little time and really get into this. Okay? Now let the experience go from your mind and spend a minute or two just paying attention to your real environment, like the furniture or whatever is around you while you're reading this. Next, recall some event that took place during the last week. Maybe a meal you had, somebody you met or a place you visited. Let that go and recall the spacecraft experience. Don't try to reconstruct it; just recall it like you did the event from last week. Let it go and recall last week's event again. Now the spacecraft once more. By now you should start to realize that—*as memories* —there really isn't any difference between the two. One might be a little more vivid in your mind than the other, but in terms of quality, both are identical. The spacecraft exercise is now indelibly recorded in your memory banks and you can recall it at will just like any other event in your life. As far as your subconscious is concerned, you have ridden in a spacecraft, and that is now part of your life experience. In fact, your subconscious probably considers it to be more "real" than many other experiences that you barely paid attention to.

Exercises

Since imagination is one of the most important tools used in creating your own reality, it will be to your advantage to develop it. Everyone has imagination, just as everyone has muscles. Both can be developed for more skillful application, so here are some imagination exercises for you to try.

Exercise 1: On a clear space in front of you, either on the floor, on the ground, or on a table, create the image of a three-foot (more or less) length of thick rope with a simple overhand knot tied in the middle. Make it a full, three-dimensional image as if it were really lying there in front of you. Now, with your imagination, reach out and touch the rope, getting a good feel for its weight and texture. Then, with your imaginary hands, untie the knot. Make sure you can clearly see and feel the whole process. If this is easy for you, you already have a well-developed imagination of the mime variety and you may want to go on to a square knot or a bowline. If you have trouble with the exercise, don't panic. That's what you're doing the exercise for. Just practice until it becomes easy. If you really have a hard time seeing the knot clearly, get a real piece of rope and tie a knot in it for reference's sake, and then go back to the "mime" rope.

Exercise 2: To show how well your body responds to imagination, try this exercise in the morning shortly after you get up, when your muscles are still a little stiff from sleep. First, with your knees straight, reach down to touch your toes from a standing position. If you can do that easily, attempt to touch your knuckles to the ground. If that's too easy, try to put your palms flat on the floor. If you can do *that* first thing in the morning, go on to the next exercise. Anyway, if you're still with me, make this first attempt without strain, noting how far your hands can go without your legs hurting. Now, straighten up and imagine that you are actually bending down and touching your toes (or further) and repeat this three times. Now reach down physically again. This time your hands ought to reach farther without strain, if not all the way. Use your imagination again if you want to improve your actual performance.

Exercise 3: At home, at work, or wherever you happen to be with a few spare moments, practice "adding" things to the environment. In other words, use your mime imagination to create something that isn't physically there, and

have fun with it. Here are some ideas to get you started:
- —put antlers on someone's head.
- —put a bear in a tree.
- —put flowers on philodendrons.
- —add tail fins and hood ornaments to cars.
- —(and when you think it's getting too easy) change the kinds of clothes that people are wearing.

Exercise 4: It's also important to develop your picture imagination so this exercise will help you. You can do this one either with your eyes closed or with your eyes open while looking at a blank area like a wall. Picture a tree standing in a field, and put in as much detail as you like. As soon as you get a nice, clear image, start making changes. Make a limb drop off the tree and then replace it in another spot. Change the color of the leaves. Make the grass grow higher and add or take away flowers. If there are no people or animals, put some in. If there are some, take them out. Whatever you do, practice until you can make the changes at will. Surprisingly, there are many people who find it difficult to make such changes. That's only because they aren't used to consciously controlling their mental images. This exercise will be good for them.

Exercise 5: Occasionally I run across people who say they don't think in images and that they can't picture things either in their mind or outside of it. But I have never had a case where I couldn't teach the person how to do it. I claim, therefore, that everyone can do it, but that for various reasons certain people have simply developed the habit of not doing it. For people who want to start, I've had the most success in having them begin by recalling dreams. Next we get into recalling and describing childhood experiences in colorful detail. Then we get into open-eyed projection of pleasing images onto a blank wall, until they are able to start on the previous four exercises. If this is your situation, you can develop your own program along these lines.

CHAPTER THREE

THε Tool of Motivation

Emotivation is the term I have given to the ability to consciously direct your emotions. Notice that I didn't say to control or repress them; either of those actions will always lead to trouble. You *direct* your emotions when you are able to harmlessly release undesirable emotions and choose the ones you want to have when you want to have them. I'll give you some practice exercises at the end of this chapter to help you learn how, but first I want to give you what may be some new ideas about emotions themselves.

Movements and Messages

Emotions are movements of energy through your body. We could call it life energy or biological energy, but all that matters is that they are flows of energy like any other. That's easily proven by the fact that strong emotions are always accompanied by sensations of heat and a rise in temperature. All that is happening is that some of the emotional energy is being converted into heat, which is in accord with the good old laws of physics. As a matter of fact, some of it is also converted into electricity, but that doesn't really concern us here. As far as heat goes, I just want you to realize that when someone says that they are "boiling mad" or feeling "warmly affectionate" they are not using meaningless metaphors.

There is more to emotions than just a movement of energy, however. What sets them apart from mere sensations of energy flow that everyone experiences from time to time is that they also carry messages. They could be compared to the messages carried by radio energy or the energy in telephone wires. The names we give to emotions—fear, anger, jealousy, joy, or affection—are descriptions of their message content. *The feeling itself is just excitement.* And we label that excitement according to the ideas that travel with it.

Where do the messages come from? Ideas and images are either stored in the cells of your body as memory or generated by you on the spot as a reaction to other ideas or outside circumstances. What triggers them off? Your own or other people's ideas, images, postures, movements, actions, or emotions are the triggers.

Emotions and Tension

The connection between our mind, our feelings, and our body is so obvious that it shouldn't come as any surprise to you when I say that emotions are intimately linked to muscular tension. In other words, your muscles are always involved in some way whenever you experience an emotion of any kind. Generally, the so-called "negative" emotions like anger and fear are accompanied by an increase in tension, while "positive" emotions like joy and affection are accompanied by a release of tension. There are a couple of apparent exceptions to this that I'll mention later on. At any rate, where emotions are concerned, what seems to happen is that an image or an idea in the mind generates nervous impulses that cause muscles to tense or to relax. These muscular reactions in turn create wave disturbances in the natural energy flow of our body—what we call emotions— at least whenever they intensify the same ideas and images or evoke other ones. Emotions aren't usually involved, for instance, when you get the idea of thirst and tense your muscles to reach for a glass of water. But emotions may be involved when you get the idea of thirst and you tense your muscles to reach out for a glass of water that someone is trying to take away from you. Let's do a couple of experiments now to show you the relationship between muscular tension and emotions.

Experiment 1: Sit comfortably in a chair, close your eyes, and tense all the muscles in your body while you count to fifteen. Then suddenly let all your muscles relax, keep your eyes closed, and just experience the sensations in your body. If you really pay attention, you ought to feel a warm glow, a tingly feeling, a sense of movement through your limbs, or possibly all three. This is simply to show you that muscle tension affects your body's energy flow. If you can imagine your body as a hose through which water is flowing, what you have just done is the equivalent of pinching the hose and then letting it go. What happens with the hose is that the water is held back for a moment and then rushes forward with a spurt before evening out again. A very similar thing happened with your body.

Experiment 2: Sit in a comfortable chair and consciously relax all the muscles in your body as best you can. You don't have to go through any elaborate procedure. Just say to yourself that you want all your muscles to relax and then let them do it. Then, *without allowing any of your muscles to get tense,* try to generate any kind of strong emotion. You can even use images if you want, as long as you don't tense your muscles. Try anger, try fear, try enthusiasm, anything you want, but without tension. How about that! If you have truly been able to keep your muscles from getting tense, you will have found that it is *impossible* to have a strong emotion while you are physically relaxed. You can't even get depressed if your muscles are really relaxed. This knowledge is of tremendous importance because it provides you with a key to the mastery of thoughts and feelings.

Tension and Release

Above I said that there are some apparent exceptions regarding the relationship between muscular tension and the kinds of emotions you experience, and I'd like to explain that now. First of all, please realize that muscle tension by itself is not bad for you. Without it you wouldn't be able to perform any physical activity at all. You wouldn't even be able to stand, sit, or smile. What's more, as you may have discovered from the last experiment, a certain amount of tension is involved in producing very pleasant emotions, too. Tension makes pleasant emotions possible, but what makes them pleasant is that the tension is accompanied by release. During a pleasant emotion, some muscles are tensing while others are releasing, and in short order the tensing muscles release while others tense up before releasing again. There seems to be a lot of tension involved in a high state of enthusiasm, for instance, but what is actually involved is a lot of simultaneous tension and release. In brief, the sense of pleasure is connected to the discharge of tension.

Unpleasant Emotions

Unpleasant emotions are connected to acute (extreme) tension or chronic (continuous) tension. If the tension is high enough, you may also experience pain as well, because all pain is caused by extreme or unrelieved tension. Anyway, what often happens during an emotion such as anger is that while the emotion is in progress and the muscles are tensing up, a person may decide that the emotion is bad, that it might be dangerous, that it is too unpleasant to continue with, or that it should be stopped for whatever reason. And so, instead of discharging it in some way, the person might try to stop it in its tracks by bunching up other muscles against it and holding it there. Then he just leaves the knot of muscles in place and tries his best to forget about the emotion. But the body hasn't forgotten. It can't, because the emotional message is still locked up in that knot of muscles, *and emotional messages don't dissipate until they're delivered.* The message is delivered when you become aware of it and let it play itself out. If you cut off the message by suppressing it, it will just remain there in your muscles until it is released. Going back to that hypothetical person I was talking about, the next time something makes him angry he is likely to react in the same way, so the muscles get a little tighter, the message is suppressed, and more energy gets locked up. That is the start of chronic tension. When chronic tension is suddenly released, all the blocked up messages and energy will pour out, giving the impression that the release is producing the emotions. But that is just an apparent and temporary effect, because if the release continues there will be pleasurable relief. If chronic tension is unrelieved for a long time it may produce either destructive physical symptoms or a disastrous emotional outburst.

Exterior Factors in Emotion

Emotions are generated by ideas and images in your mind, which also induce changes in muscular tension. But your ideas and images are often influenced by events and circumstances outside your body. The most obvious influence comes from the behavior of other people. If someone's behavior happens to get you emotionally upset, it is because such behavior evokes ideas and images in your mind that trigger emotions. A few minutes ago while writing this chapter I got a call from one of my young sons who was upset because his older brother was making faces at him through a window. It wasn't the fact that the older boy was making faces that got him upset, because in other circumstances I have seen the younger one laugh at such antics. What got the young one upset was that in this case he held the *idea* that the older one was making fun of him. So as much as you might like to, you can't justify blaming someone else's behavior for your emotional reactions. Your ideas and images are the more direct cause, not their behavior.

A less obvious influence comes from other people's emotions, regardless of their behavior. Besides the currents of energy flowing through our bodies, each one of us is surrounded by what can be described as an "energy field." This field contains a lot of stuff, including heat and electromagnetic radiation, gaseous chemicals discharged from your cells and your breath, and the same life energy that runs through your body. The nature and content of this field changes according to your emotional state, and it is also influenced by your mental images and ideas. In addition, this field is influenced by other people's fields and by their images and ideas. For all practical purposes we can call it an "emotional field" because it carries the message content of your images and ideas. Actually, a better term would be "emotional atmosphere" since it accurately reflects your inner climate, from storms to clear weather.

You can sense or feel other people's emotions through this atmosphere no matter what their behavior even when you can't see them. Of course, some people are much more sensitive to this emotional field than others, just as some are more sensitive to weather, but nearly everyone can sense the "charged" atmosphere of a room in which strong emotions are operating regardless of whether the people are trying to put on a polite front. And many people can sense the same atmosphere after those who generated it have left. Also, when you are around someone who is experiencing strong emotions, those emotions will tend to awaken and intensify corresponding or associated ideas and images in your mind which then will tend to evoke similar emotions in yourself. Often people will go half out of their minds trying to discover the cause within themselves for a sudden attack of anxiety, sadness, or whatever when the triggering factor was really the emotional state of someone else. I've experienced this in my own office. I'd be thinking everything was fine until an emotionally upset employee started to work in the next room, and within a few minutes I'd start to become irritable for no apparent reason. Distance isn't very important in this kind of thing, as many mothers of small children can attest. It is possible to experience "emotional empathy" with a person quite far away from you. This is most common between close relatives, especially twins and intimate companions, but it may happen even between casual friends. Once I was working quietly all alone when I suddenly began to feel anxious and got a sudden urge to check the want ads for a job. On the face of it this was silly, but the urge was strong. Within a half hour a friend called to tell me he had lost his job that morning and wanted me to help him find another one. The main reason I responded to his feeling was that at the time my job was new and I was feeling insecure about it. The point to remember is that emotions from other people can't affect you unless you have a corresponding or associated idea running around somewhere in your own head. At the end of the chapter I will give you a technique for protecting yourself against unwanted empathy.

Just for the record, there are a few physical conditions that can affect your emotions, too. The lack of certain vitamins and minerals, particularly the B vitamins and calcium, may add to your emotional instability and supplements could help. The lack itself, though, was probably brought about by stress-related thinking in the first place. In such a case you should supplement your thinking as well as your body. Atmospheric ionization is another factor, and so is the variation in solar and lunar gravity. This book isn't the place to go into such factors, but they, too, affect you only according to your conscious and unconscious ideas about yourself and your world.

Emotional Mastery

With this brief background on the effects of emotions recapped, it's time to return to emotivation. As I said at the beginning of the chapter, *emotivation is the ability to consciously direct your emotions* instead of letting them push you around. Now I'll describe some of the common techniques for doing this.

Deep breathing is probably the most basic technique used for emotional mastery. Generally, the more emotionally agitated a person is, the more shallow and rapid their breathing becomes. This is because of the increasing tension. Slow, deep breathing tends to counteract the tension and even-out the flow of energy, so the agitation quickly fades away. It is important that the breathing be *slow,* or you might get dizzy. After the deep breathing calms you down you can make clearer decisions about your reactions.

Sublimation is an old stand-by technique still popular in the human potential movement. It simply refers to expressing your unpleasant or undesirable emotions in acceptable ways. Rolling up a newspaper and beating a table instead of your boss' head is an example. Screaming out your feelings while alone in your car (with the windows rolled up, please!) works well, too. Another excellent alternative is banging out your thoughts and feelings on a typewriter in descriptive detail. Who knows? You might even produce a best-seller. In sublimation, you aren't trying to change the emotions. What you are doing is using ideas and images to influence your actions and change the means of expression.

Redirection or transformation involves the use of ideas and images to transform one emotion into another. Normally, when an idea or image triggers an emotional flow, the emotion tends to reinforce the idea or image, which restimulates the emotion, and back and forth they go. In redirection, you consciously change the idea or image without stopping the flow, so that only the message content is changed. A friend of mine recently told me how she did this with fear. She was embarking on a new enterprise and was full of fearful emotions. Being acquainted with the idea of emotions as energy, she changed her ideas and images of possible failure into ideas and images of an adventure into the unknown, and thus transformed the fear into anticipatory excitement. This technique works well with long-standing habitual emotions.

Emotional inducement is a means of using ideas and images to generate an emotion where one is apparently lacking. I say 'apparently' because apathy or boredom is essentially a fear response, and depression is a form of suppressed anger. Indifference, procrastination, laziness, and the like can all serve as emotional disguises that keep us from doing the things we want to do. Since ideas and images are what stimulate emotions, emotional inducement consists of deliberately choosing ideas and images that tend to produce strongly active emotional responses, and then carrying out an associated action. One of the most arousing emotions is anger, and this is sometimes a good antidote to emotional lethargy. As someone once said, an angry man can accomplish miracles. But this refers to expressed anger and, specifically, righteous anger directed to correcting wrongs. The ideas and images you use have to incite you to action, not just trap you on a merry-go-round of ill-feelings. Once action has been initiated, the ideas and images can be modified to redirect the anger into enthusiasm for accomplishing good, rather than merely correcting wrongs. An alternative to anger as an emotional inducement is compassion for others. I have seen cases where boredom and depression have disappeared like magic when a person's interest was directed toward helping others resolve their problems. Inducing emotions on your own is not easy, however, and it is generally more effective when you have a friend to help you focus on the new ideas and images that are necessary.

Emotional observation is a technique that requires practice, because it involves letting your emotions flow without any suppression and without letting them goad you into any undesirable or ineffective action. It means, first of all, that you have to recognize emotions for what they really are—message-carrying streams of energy, and nothing more. You have to stop identifying with them and establish a sort of detached, "well-look-what's-happening" attitude. A helpful way to start is to get out of the habit of saying something like "I am angry" and get into the habit of saying "I am feeling anger," which is a more true statement anyway. When you can feel emotions without *being* them, you can start paying attention to what they are saying. By watching the thoughts that arise in your mind during the emotion you can discover the ideas and images on which it is based. When the emotion has run its course you can then decide to change those images and ideas.

Another technique that needs practice is conscious muscular relaxation. It requires that you learn to pay attention to your body, especially the degree of tension in your muscles. With practice you can become aware of the tension simultaneously with the build-up of emotion. Then you can consciously relax your muscles and allow the emotional energy to dissipate. This way you can get the message without the reaction, and for this reason it works very well in conjunction with emotional observation. You should realize that the energy doesn't just disappear. It simply spreads throughout your body as pure energy, and is available for redirection.

Exercises

Here are a few practice exercises to help train your emotivational abilities.

Exercise 1: This is a deep breathing exercise that many of my students have found to be extremely effective. You'll get the greatest benefit from it by using it before meeting with other people when you want to remain calm, just after an emotional outburst when you are still feeling unpleasant effects, and whenever you are alone and feeling nervous or upset.

Sit comfortably and place your hands in your lap, either with your palms up or with the fingertips of each hand touching. Let out your breath and do the following:

1. Breathe in and repeat the word "Release, release, release, release."
2. Hold your breath in while mentally saying, "Release, release, release, release."
3. Let your breath out to the word "Relax, relax, relax, relax."
4. Hold your breath as you repeat "Relax, relax, relax, relax."
5. Do the above four times in all, and *do it slowly*. After the last time, just breathe naturally.

I have an alternative set of words that produces a slightly different effect, if you like. In this case you do your breathing to the words "One ringy-dingy, two ringy-dingies, three ringy-dingies, four ringy-dingies." Try it. Unless you are severely upset, you may find yourself laughing at the absurdity of it before you have finished, and laughter is the best tension reliever of all.

Exercise 2: This is an exercise to help you realize the power of images in influencing your emotions. First, list in separate columns the various emotions, including what you consider to be negative ones as well as positive ones. Then, opposite each one you've listed, briefly describe a scene or an incident from your memory that most closely corresponds to the emotion listed. To make the exercise easier, list the positive and negative emotions on separate pieces of paper. Now find a quiet spot, pick out one of the negative emotions, and let your picture imagination dwell on the related scene or incident until you start to feel the related emotion welling up. As soon as the emotion is on its way, pick one of the positive emotions and dwell on that related scene or incident until the new emotion starts welling up. Go back and forth among the emotions and memories until you have gone through the whole list, making sure that you have finished up on a positive emotion. Be aware during the whole process how the emotions respond to the images on which you focus. Through this kind of direct experience you will quickly learn how you do and can use your mind to direct your feelings. Pick out a few of your favorite scenes or incidents, those that evoke the strongest positive emotions, and put them on a special card that you can carry with you and refer to until they are quickly available for recall. Then, whenever negative emotions are starting to get you down, remember one of these scenes or incidents and dwell on it until your mood has changed and you can go back and deal with the cause of the previous emotion. Use this as a means of clearing your energy system, not as an escape mechanism for avoiding what you have to deal with.

Exercise 3: This simple exercise is to help you learn indirect control of your emotions through muscular relaxation. Get in a comfortable position and practice tensing and releasing every muscle in your body. Start with your head, practicing tension/ release with your forehead, your eyes, your cheeks, your mouth, etc., going slowly and carefully all the way down to your toes. You don't have to tense your muscles very much; just enough so that you can feel them when you release. Pay close attention, because through this exercise you want to learn what your muscles feel like when they are tensed and how they feel when they are relaxed, and then what it feels like to make the change. In this way you will become more aware of what your muscles are doing in the course of your daily activities, especially those involving confrontations with other people, and you will be able to release unwanted tension before it has a chance to build up. It is a good idea, too, to learn to notice what you or others are saying or doing or what is occurring when your muscles tense up. That will give you a powerful clue to responsive ideas and images that you may want to change.

Exercise 4: This last exercise in emotivation involves the establishment of what I call a "mind-shield." It actually consists of using your mime imagination to set up a shield of light that completely surrounds you. There are many possible variations of this, but I recommend imagining a halo over the top of your head, and then streams of pleasantly colored light, like sunbeams pouring down from the edges of the halo all around you. You can use any color you want to, but most of the people I've worked with find gold or pink to be best. To make it more effective, perform Exercise 1 just before you do this one for the first few times. While in that relaxed state, imagine the shield and say something like "This shield is protecting me from all undesirable influences; only that which is good for me can come through." Thereafter, all you will have to do is take one deep breath, say the word "Shield!" and imagine it there. The purpose of this mental shield is to give you emergency protection from the effects of other people's emotional fields. Since ideas and images affect emotions and behavior, the idea and image of this shield will affect your emotional and physical responses so that you will be less susceptible to the emotions of others. After some practice, I suggest using the shield whenever you get a sudden attack of unreasonable anxiety or other undesirable emotion, and even when you get a sudden, inexplicable pain. If these are merely the effects of someone else's problems, they will quickly diminish or disappear. If the shield doesn't work after you have practiced with it for awhile, then you know you have to look within for the source. If you are not already familiar with mind-shielding, I think you will be in for some pleasant surprises, especially when dealing with people who habitually get you emotionally upset.

CHAPTER FOUR

THE Tool of CONCENTRATION

Concentration is nothing more than sustained attention. It just means keeping your mind on one thing to the exclusion of other things. It's a tool you are already familiar with because you use it in many activities, such as reading an interesting book, watching a good movie or television program, or being deeply involved in a hobby or project. When you are concentrating all your attention on what you are doing, you are likely to be oblivious to what else is going on around you, including people calling you to dinner. It is your interest in something that determines how well you can concentrate on it. Concentration and interest (or you could call it motivation) go hand-in-hand. So one general rule for concentration is: The more you like or are interested in something, the easier it is to concentrate on it; the less you like or the less interested you are in something, the harder it is to concentrate on it.

Children have incredible powers of concentration. If you doubt this, try calling a kid who is playing an exciting game to tell him it's time to clean up his room. Short of physical force or shouting in his ear, it may be almost impossible to break his concentration. Seriously, the child may not be consciously ignoring your call. He has just tuned out anything less interesting than the game. Usually, when we say a child can't concentrate, we mean he *won't* concentrate on what we want him to. But they do an excellent job of concentration when it involves something of interest to them. Just for the sake of science, after unsuccessfully trying to break my youngest son's concentration while he was playing a game, I once went to a patio door two rooms away. In an ordinary voice I said to my wife who was outside, "I wonder if any of the kids would like a dollar?" Immediately came a young voice from the game room, "I do!" This gives rise to another axiom: Concentration tends to be automatically directed toward areas of greatest personal concern or interest.

What Makes Concentration Hard

Most people seem to have grown up with the idea that concentration is hard work, that it takes a lot of effort to do. If I were to ask you to give me an image of someone in deep concentraton, it's quite likely that you would describe someone with a tightened mouth and a frown. The impression would be of someone struggling to do something he really didn't want to do. I suspect that this stereotype stems from our school days when we were told to concentrate on our studies instead of the many other things we would have preferred to do. But, as I have already said, you are concentrating whenever your attention is directed to one thing for more than a few moments. You might be inclined to ask where I draw the line between mere attention and the sustained attention called concentration. Well, the line is a fine one, but just so we can have a clear concept to work with, I am going to arbitrarily define concentration as attention directed toward any one thing for longer than thirty seconds. You think that sounds too easy? Then try the following:

Experiment: Take a picture from a magazine or one you might have on the wall, and direct your attention to it for one minute. So that you can keep your mind on what you are doing, you may want to have a friend do the timing or use a kitchen timer. Next, pick the smallest object you can find in that picture and direct your full attention to it for one minute, without paying any attention to the rest of the picture and without thinking any unrelated thoughts. What you will find after doing this is that keeping your attention on the whole picture was pretty easy, but that keeping it on the one object was more difficult. We can get some other axioms about concentration from this: The greater the field of focus (that is, the more things there are to catch your attention), the easier it is to concentrate; and the smaller the field of focus (that is, the fewer things there are to hold your attention), the more difficult it is to concentrate. You may also have experienced still another axiom: The harder you think it is to concentrate, the harder it becomes.

Now, concentration makes a very valuable mental tool because it produces some curious effects that we can make practical use of. Three of the main effects will be described in the next sections.

The Altered State Effect

The brain is a magnificent living computer designed to process an immense amount of information from many sources. When its habitual sources of information from the world around us are restricted through a narrowing of attention for more than a few moments (concentration), it tends to shift to another mode of functioning. When this happens, more information is extracted from a given focus of attention than would ordinarily be the case, or else information is sought out from non-habitual sources. This different mode or way of functioning is called nowadays an "altered state of consciousness," and it includes such things as hypnotic trance, various meditative states, and even ordinary sleep. Daydreaming is an altered state, too, and some people go into altered states of consciousness while reading or watching TV. If you have ever been reading a book and suddenly realized that you have no idea of what you read for the past few paragraphs or pages, then you've experienced this yourself.

All over the world, people of many different times and cultures have consciously induced this effect in order to experience various forms of altered states for a number of reasons, including health. All the techniques center around holding a narrow focus of attention until the brain "shifts gears," so to speak. The most common ways to do this are to concentrate on a single physical object (like a flower or a piece of crystal) or drawing (especially a geometrical pattern); to concentrate on a static or monotonous image in the mind; or to concentrate on repetitive words or musical rhythms.

To be most effective, the concentration has to be narrowed to the point where you don't even analyze what you are concentrating on — you just "experience" it. This is exactly what you do when you go to sleep. You narrow your range of conscious focus until your brain shifts over to another kind of awareness. This same effect is what's behind the old prescription to count sheep in order to fall asleep. The monotonous regularity of the sheep jumping over the stile causes the brain to shift gears. Doing multiplication tables can achieve the same end. The problem with most insomniacs is that they keep their brain busy by thinking about a lot of different subjects in scattered order, analyzing, judging, evaluating, projecting, etc. The cure is simply to keep the mind focused on one thing, whether it be a spot on the wall, an image in the mind, or a piece of music like Ravel's "Bolero." However, while sleep is definitely therapeutic, many health benefits can be obtained during types of altered states in which you remain awake.

The Informational Flow Effect

Here is another axiom for you: Concentration on a given idea or image tends to stimulate corresponding ideas, images, or insights. In this context, let's say that an insight is an idea or image which gives you information you hadn't thought of before.

In order to achieve this effect, your concentration has to be a little less restricted than for the altered state effect.

The technique is to hold the idea or image in your mind while at the same time allowing thoughts about it to enter your awareness. Creative scientists, inventors, writers, and artists use this a lot. For a while it was quite popular in the business world under the name of "brainstorming," a process whereby a problem was presented and a group of people spewed out solutions as fast as they could think of them, without regard to how silly or crazy they sounded. The concept was that the more ideas that were allowed to flow without restriction, the greater was the likelihood that some of them would be practical, even if unorthodox.

The informational flow effect is good for creative inspiration and problem solving, but that's not all. It is also good for achieving greater understanding of whatever you are concentrating on. In ancient times this was the primary means of scientific and philosophical investigation of nature, and it had the advantage of not requiring the destruction of life in order to study it. It is somewhat of a "lost art" today, practiced by very few although still available to all. The best example I can think of where this effect was used in modern times was by Luther Burbank, the "Wizard of Horticulture." Burbank was quoted in *The Secret Life of Plants* (Tompkins & Bird) as saying that his art was basically "a matter of concentration and the rapid elimination of nonessentials." And he produced all his wonders without a laboratory.

The Reproduction Effect

I think this effect is the most important one of all, as well as the most curious, the most common, and the most difficult to believe when you first hear about it. It is based on the following axiom: Concentration on a given idea or image tends to reproduce the nearest equivalent in physical experience. In other words, the kinds of thoughts you dwell on are what determine to a large extent your experience of life. Or, to put it still another way, the circumstances you find yourself in and the events you experience are reflections of your most persistent thoughts. Let me assure you that this is not a case of mystical symbology, but it is a demonstrable fact. Strangely enough, this is one of mankind's oldest teachings, and yet hardly anyone seems to take it seriously. If more people did, they wouldn't be blaming their parents, society, television, God or anyone else for their present situations. How it actually works is still an open question, though there are any number of theories ranging from telepathic attraction to unconsciously induced motivation, but let's leave theories aside. The main point is that it does work and you can prove it to yourself through practice.

The kind of concentration it takes is that in which you hold an idea or image strongly and clearly in your mind without analyzing it, but without letting it shift you into another state of awareness either. I've found that mime imagination works best for this because it tends to keep you focused in the full waking state. Picture imagination can be used, but it tends to take longer to produce physical effects and it also tends to lead more easily to altered states or informational flow. Specific ways to use this for healing will be brought out in Part II of this book, but for now I'll just give you a couple of examples from my own experience to show you what can occur.

On one occasion I attended a conference at a big hotel, and when I left I found I had forgotten a valuable briefcase. When I went back it was nowhere in sight, so I left word with the management to look for it. I called the next day and they said they had found it, but when I went back it turned out to be someone else's. I asked them to keep looking, but they didn't have much hope of finding it after two days. At this point I could have just kicked myself and given up, but I got angry and refused to accept the apparent fact that it was lost. For the next two days I *vividly* imagined the briefcase in my possession and absolutely cancelled any doubts that I would get it back. Then I called the hotel again and was told that they had it. It was sitting in plain view in a place that had already been checked by the staff and myself. Did it materialize out of thin air? Most probably not. Was it a coincidence? Well, my students and myself have too many successes with this effect for us to believe in coincidences any more.

Now, depending partly on circumstances and partly on your intentions, the reproduction effect usually brings into your experience *the nearest available equivalent* to your image first. That equivalent could be something resembling your image, a picture of it, somebody talking about it, or the same thing in someone else's possession or experience. For instance, I once imaged ten thousand dollars in my hot little hands so well I could feel the bills. Within a few days I found myself in a position where I had to withdraw ten thousand in cash from a bank for an organization I was working for. I had the money in my hot little hands, but it wasn't mine. On another occasion I was thinking about this effect and idly imaged something far out — a blue carnation — just to see what would happen. Four days later my wife told me a story about a man who always gave his wife blue-tinted carnations on her birthday to match her eyes.

Three days or more seems to be an average gestation period for this effect to take place, though many times it will happen more quickly. Whether or not the image becomes reproduced as part of your personal experience and/or possession depends a lot on the intensity of your imaging, your intent to have it happen, and your persistence. The Reproduction Effect of concentration is an exceptionally worthwhile part of your mental toolkit for healing.

Exercises

The following practice exercises will help train you in several forms of concentration.

Exercise 1: On a piece of white paper, draw a concentric circle or spiral with about seven turns, one to two inches in diameter. Don't be bothered if it isn't perfect. While seated comfortably and alone, hold the paper and simply gaze at the spiral for about five minutes (a timer isn't necessary). Feel free to blink and lower your eyelids almost closed if you want to. The less you think about anything the better, but don't try to force your thinking to stop. Let any thoughts drift by while you hold your attention gently on the spiral. After five minutes or so, close your eyes and let your mind drift while you observe your own sensations of sight, sound and feeling. Open your eyes whenever you feel like it.

What this exercise will do is to quickly put you in an altered state of consciousness where you may have some interesting experiences. While gazing at the spiral, it may seem to move and you may seem to see wavelike and flashing movements across its surface. You might also sense sudden movements in your peripheral vision, and a tingling, numbness and/or great sense of relaxation in your body. A hissing or ringing sound might also appear. When you close your eyes you may see colored lights and shapes, and you may experience dream-like sequences of events. Your senses are not playing "tricks" on you. It's just that you have shifted your awareness so that you perceive data that you normally ignore. Of course, you may have a totally different experience than I've described, you may experience nothing at all, or you may even fall asleep. If you experience nothing, you need more practice. If you fall asleep, you need more rest.

Exercise 2: For this exercise, pick a "big" topic like Life, Love, Money, Friendship, Sex, Joy, Power, Health or anything that interests you and is of potential concern to others. Relax in a comfortable position and ask yourself, "What is _____?" Then let your thoughts revolve around the topic for five to ten minutes. What you are trying to achieve is a sort of inner conversation, in which images enhance the conversation but do not replace it. If the inner conversation seems to run down, stimulate it with further questions like, "What else is it?" or "Why do I think that about it?" and "What do other people think about it and why?"

This is a real test of concentration, because unless you are used to focusing on one idea in an open-minded way for any length of time you are likely to find your mind quickly "jumping the track" to think about anything but the topic you've chosen. If this happens, just gently bring your attention back to the main idea as soon as you notice you've gotten away from it. This exercise can be considered successful when you have received a new insight about the topic in question, or when you have recalled something important and positive about it that you had forgotten.

Exercise 3: This one is used to practice awareness of the Reproduction Effect of concentration. All you have to do is pick a fairly unusual object to concentrate on. Some examples to get you thinking could be a $100 bill, a Model-T Ford, a dragon, a white elephant, a blue rose, or whatever. Then get comfortable and, using mime imagination, visualize that object in front of you as clearly and in as much sensory detail as you can for five full minutes. You will find it easier to hold the image if you either see it in motion (like the elephant walking) or if you "pulse" the image (visualize it strongly and let it fade, and repeat that over and over). If you have concentrated well, that object will *in some fashion* appear in your environment. I suggest that you give it at least three days, though it could be a little shorter or longer. When it does appear, you will feel a wonderful shock of pleasure and surprise. It will be your first convincing proof of the power of mind over matter.

CHAPTER FIVE

The Tool of Affirmation

"To affirm" means to make a positive, confident statement. I call it a mental tool because it takes conscious decision and will, and because such statements represent ideas that affect emotions, behavior, and health. Although you can make affirmative statements to or about other people, I am referring here to ones you make to or about yourself. This is something you do all the time, but I want to help you be more conscious of it so that it really does become a tool, instead of a semi-conscious habit.

Affirmative statements are usually thought of in terms of words, but your posture and gestures can also be affirmations in a way. In the next two sections I will discuss both verbal and postural affirmations.

Affirmative Speech

The ideas we hold about ourselves or about various aspects of life are often expressed through our speech patterns. By a "speech pattern" I don't mean the way we talk, but the habitual words or phrases we use to describe ourselves and our feelings. It frequently happens that the use of these words has become such a habit that we don't even realize it when we are saying them. I have conversed with many people who assure me how positive they are, even when their life is a mess. But in the course of the conversation they will usually let slip something that contradicts their positiveness and shows why they are in such straits. When I call them on it, they quite often don't even remember having said it. Yet, those "unconscious" statements have more effect on their life than all the carefully planned positive ones, precisely because they are habitual. If such statements are brought to their attention they might say something like, "Well, I didn't really mean that, it was just an expression. What I really believe is . . . " Sorry, but that just doesn't hold water. We all have the curious ability to control our speech so that we say things that sound good, that we think we "should" believe. However, they may not correspond at all to the ideas that are actually operating within us. That's why it is the spontaneous words and phrases we use that reveal our true feelings and beliefs. Their very spontaneity classes them as operating habits.

Some of you may already be familiar with the idea of affirmations, but there's a difference between *effective affirmations* and nice-sounding statements that just come off the top of your head. For one thing, many recommended affirmations are either too long or too vague. Long and rambling affirmations have virtually no effect on behavior, though they may give you a temporary good feeling. The subconscious part of your mind, which is directly involved in your state of health, reacts much better to statements that are short and to the point. For instance, here is a typical long-winded, well-intentioned affirmation:

> The Healing Power of the Universe which is unlimited and eternal is flowing into every part of my body, filling me with Light and Peace and Health. I know that this is so and I accept the abundant well-being and vitality that it brings and I give thanks for the bountiful blessings of good health that result.

I have seen some of these go on for pages. By contrast, a simple statement like "My body is healing now!" said over and over will achieve much better results, even though it might be less intellectually satisfying.

An effective affirmation also needs to be specific enough to have clear meaning for you. If the meaning is vague, then the results will be vague, too. Many years ago a man named Emile Coué promoted a nice short affirmation that went "Every day in every way I am getting better and better." Such an affirmation would only have a positive effect if you were very clear in your mind as to what "better" meant for you. It's basically a good phrase, though, and you can modify it to suit your aims by subsituting more specific words for "better and better."

Affirmations work best when they deal with changing ideas that you hold about yourself or about life in general. After all, the ideas you've been holding got you 'where you're at.' The trick is to learn to catch yourself when you're using a phrase that could produce negative effects. If you find yourself saying something like "I'm always sick at this time of year," then stop and say to yourself "Change that!" And replace the negative with something like "I'm always healthy," even if you only say it to yourself.

By the way, some nonsense has been written about affirmations to the effect that "You should never use a negative statement like 'I never get sick' because your subconscious doesn't hear negatives." The idea is that your subconscious would only hear "I get sick." Well, let me tell you that your subconscious hears everything you say. Nevertheless, I do recommend purely positive statements because it is too easy for an image of sickness to pop up when you say "I never get sick." And your subconscious sees all the images you produce, too.

Besides being short, clear, specific, and positive, a good affirmation is also one you believe, at least a little bit. If an affirmation goes directly against your beliefs it will take a long time for it to start having positive effects, if it ever does. As an example, if you are seriously ill, it won't do you much good to go around saying "I am perfectly healthy" because that would probably be too far removed from your existing reality to be effective in changing your condition. Your subconscious mind just wouldn't accept it. But if you changed the wording to "I *can* be perfectly healthy" it becomes more believable, and therefore more effective. On the other hand, if you are already pretty healthy then "I can be perfectly healthy" could be meaningless unless you had a specific idea about what perfect health means to you. One way to get around that is to say "I can be healthier than I am." In any case, the magic phrase in many affirmations is "I CAN." As long as you believe it's *possible* for you to be or do what you want, the statement will work, once you've established it as a habitual thought pattern.

Habits are formed by repetition. The repetition first takes place in the mind, with images and ideas, and then it gives rise to habitual emotions, speech, and behavior. Now, it happens to be a fact of human nature that the only way to get rid of an old habit is to replace it with a new one. Even if you stop smoking, what you have done is to substitute a nonsmoking habit for a smoking one. Habitual words and phrases are like constant reinforcers that either limit thought and action or allow them to expand. The purpose of affirmations is to help you consciously develop the kind of habitual reinforcement you give yourself.

Here are some exercises to work with.

Exercise 1: Throughout the course of a day, pay close attention to the self-limiting words and phrases that people use about themselves. Look for such things as "I can't...I always...I never..." as well as words that they use to belittle themselves. See if you can relate what they say about themselves to the way their lives are working.

Exercise 2: This is a little harder. Throughout the course of a day, pay close attention to your own self-limiting words and phrases, particularly when you are talking about those areas of your life in which you may have difficulty. Make a list of them and see how you may be reinforcing the very things you don't like.

Exercise 3: Particularly when you are feeling tired or ill, pay attention to how many times you reinforce the condition by telling someone about it. Practice feeling the way you feel without telling anyone, and instead affirm to yourself that you are or are going to get better.

Exercise 4: Pick out the most negative statement you find yourself making about yourself or your life on a habitual basis, change it to a believable affirmation, then use imagination, emotivation, and concentration with the statement for a whole month and observe whatever improvements result.

Affirmative Posture

You may have heard of the term "body language." It refers to the way we unconsciously use our body to convey our inner feelings as well as our ideas about ourselves and the world. I will be going into this in much greater detail in Part II, but for now I just want to say that posture is a form of behavior. Ideas affect behavior, and behavior can influence and stimulate ideas. When I speak of posture, I am including our gestures and all the ways we hold our bodies under varying circumstances. By changing your posture in an affirmative way you can reinforce positive ideas and emotions.

If you want to reinforce ideas of strength, friendliness, health, vitality, and self-confidence, you can practice standing and moving your limbs in ways that make you feel more of those qualities. Positive ideas, of course, will influence your posture automatically. Recently I saw a girl become literally transformed while making positive affirmations about herself. She was a decent-looking girl, but she thought of herself as much plainer than she was. In the course of an exercise she had to repeat over and over "I am beautiful." Before she started her body was slouched and she looked like she was cringing in fear. After a few moments, while making the statement, she unconsciously straightened her shoulders, lifted her head, and began to "glow." It looked like magic, but all it was, was her body's reaction to the affirmation.

Changing the posture alone won't do the whole job. It is an excellent added reinforcer, but you can't change ideas just by changing your posture: All that will do is make you a good actor. Not long ago I read of a famous actor whom everyone thought was always super cool, calm, and collected because that was how he looked. But in an interview he admitted that he was almost always a nervous wreck and he had adopted the right kind of posture to hide that.

Used in combination with affirmative speech and positive intent, however, postural affirmation helps to establish new ideas and habits more quickly and permanently.

Exercise 1: Look at yourself in a full-length mirror, from the front and the sides. Just stand normally. Do you think your posture conveys an impression of self-confidence, health, and vitality? Or do you look beaten down, scared, and weak? Change your posture so that you look heroic. How does that feel? Think about the reasons why, they may reveal some of your ideas about yourself that you haven't faced.

Exercise 2: The next time you are with a group of people, either friends or strangers, pay attention to the way you automatically position your arms, hands and legs. Do you think your positions are open or defensive? Try changing them to the opposite of whatever they are. How does that make you feel? Think about why you hold yourself the way you do, and realize it may be saying something about your feelings toward others.

Exercise 3: Pick a quality that you wish to cultivate. Self-confidence is a good one to start with. In front of a mirror, stand and move as if you were really as self-confident as you would like to be. For the next month, practice this posture when you are with people you know. Don't tell anyone what you are doing, and don't over dramatize. You don't want to come on like a prima donna or a ham. Just be aware of acting self-confident when you sit, stand or move. Watch how others react and how you begin to feel about yourself.

CHAPTER SIX

A Short Tour of Your Mind

To aid you in understanding yourself, your thoughts, and your behavior, I want to give you a way of looking at your mind — a practical way that many have found very useful. Don't worry about whether it conforms to what you may have been taught. The mind is such a multi-dimensional wonder that any system for dividing it into parts is only an arbitrary convenience. Your mind is actually an unlimited whole with a great diversity of functions. But because of that diversity, sometimes it *is* convenient to divide it into categories so that we can make better use of it.

For convenience's sake, then, let's divide the mind into three categories according to function. I'll call these the Creative Mind, the Directing Mind, and the Active Mind. In practical terms, we can say that these three categories of Mind form a cooperative venture which allows you to experience life. Sometimes that cooperation isn't very good, though. When that happens, life itself doesn't seem to be very good. Usually the problem is that we are trying to make one of these Minds function in a way it wasn't designed to do. And that is about as effective as trying to make the liver pump blood, or have the heart digest our food. What we need is a clear idea of the function of each Mind so that the cooperation will be effective.

The Creative Mind

This part of your mind is also called the Higher Self, the god-self, Spirit, the Guardian Angel, and other terms intended to convey its basic nature. It isn't God, in the sense of the Ultimate Being, but it is the part of you that most directly knows God or Universal Mind, and which acts as your channel for the power of life. Essentially, its function is to present you with knowledge, to sustain your physical existence, to supply you with "life force" and to act as sort of an agent of God in creating your individual experience by using the patterns of your thoughts.

You are not a stranger to this part of your mind, the Creative, regardless of what you may think. It is not something you have to struggle to attain. You do not have to "purify" yourself in order to experience it. It is a natural part of your daily life. Your Creative Mind is always operating with you, but you may not always be aware of it. And those times when you have been aware of it, you may not have recognized it for what it was. Below are some of the instances when your Creative Mind is in the forefront of your experience:

1. When you "know" something suddenly with a quiet, sure knowledge that is free from doubts and logic.
2. When you are quietly aware of a person, an object or an event as a "pure experience" without judgments, analysis, or inner conversation about it.
3. When you feel a part of yourself "standing apart" and quietly observing whatever you are doing.
4. When you are aware of being "at one" with nature, and you feel the quiet joy that comes with that realization.

How can you make practical use of this part of your mind? Here are three ways. First, remind yourself frequently that your Creative Mind creates your experience by using your thoughts as patterns. It doesn't use every thought, of course. Just those that you dwell on mostly. And the process is virtually automatic. What you have to do is to remember that it is happening and that the rest of you doesn't need to do anything except to take advantage of opportunities as they arise and to keep your thoughts on the kind of life or conditions that you really want to experience. The second way is to communicate with this part of your mind by mentally asking for solutions to problems that confront you or for extra energy or for strength and health. Your Creative Mind knows all the answers and it has an unlimited supply of life-giving energy, but it has the curious trait of never interfering with your free will. So, apart from basic maintenance and support, you have to ask for more help before you get it. The third way is to cultivate an awareness of this part of your mind by simple exercises. Here are a couple you can use.

Exercise 1: For this one you need nature's help. Find a place with a view where you can sit for awhile. The length of time doesn't matter; it can range from a few moments to hours. Use the beach, a lake, the woods, a garden, sunrise or sunset, wherever it is convenient. If you are severely limited in your access to nature, use a potted plant or flower, or, as a last resort (which can work very well), use a beautiful photograph of a natural setting. Spend your time just being aware of the beauty and the wonder of the life within the scene, and of the same kind of life within yourself. Let any other thoughts just drift past and fade away. Focus on the present moment, the present experience. You will finish feeling refreshed, relaxed, and clear. Think about the fact that the beautiful experience was your creation, too.

Exercise 2: Imagine your Creative Mind as a halo floating just above your head, like the kind that angels wear in comic strips. See it as glowing with a soft light and know that it is always there as a source of knowledge and strength. You have already used this halo in one of the Emotivation exercises. As an alternative, imagine your Creative Mind as a gigantic person, massive as the earth itself and able to reach up to the stars, a person who cares deeply for you and even holds you in its arms. In either form, be aware of its presence as a supportive part of yourself that wants only what is best for you. Do this when you get up in the morning and during the day whenever you think of it. The more you do this, the more you pay attention to the fact that this part of your mind exists, the more it will operate in your favor.

The Directing Mind

If you are like practically every other human being, you are probably most familiar with this part of your mind. Sometimes it is called the Conscious Mind, the Reasoning Mind or the Intellect, but those terms don't adequately describe its function. Its "job" is to take raw information from your sensations and feelings and give it meaning; to analyze and organize that information; to provide guidelines in the form of ideas and images for the Creative Mind to work with; and to give orders to the Active Mind. The last two functions have the most direct bearing on your experience of life, for it can be said that the Creative Mind brings about events and circumstances while the Active Mind generates your behavioral responses to those events and circumstances. Both, however, do their thing according to the "policies" (ideas, images and orders) of the Directing Mind.

Do you realize what I'm saying? It is that YOU are the source of your experience. The kind of person you are, the kind of work you do, where you live, the people who are prominent in your life, the nature of your relationships, your sense of happiness or unhappiness — all of these have their origin in the ideas, images, decisions and orders of your Directing Mind. What about your childhood, you may say? What about your place of birth, your parents, your race, your early environment? Surely these didn't have their origin in this Directing Mind? You're right, they didn't. The time, place, and circumstances of your birth and early years had another, higher source. But from the moment you made your first interpretation, your first analysis, your first organization of facts, or your first decision *about* the world you were born into, then your Directing Mind began its work. Well, you might say, what about my parents, my teachers and friends? They played a big role in shaping my life, didn't they? Of course they did. But their role was and is limited to being part of your experience. They may have exerted an influence, but you are still the one who made the interpretations and decisions about that influence. And those ideas and their related images are what guide your life.

The difficulties that most people have with their Directing Mind are that they either over use it, under use it, or misuse it.

You *over* use it by worrying about past or present situations that you either can't change or have no control over, by constantly analyzing and judging, by giving things more meaning than they deserve, and by making decisions based on your emotions.

You *under* use it by pretending that you are at the mercy of your habits, by allowing yourself to get locked into a dull and joyless routine of living, and by refusing to think about what you can do to make life better for yourself.

You *misuse* it by blaming others for your circumstances, by making up all kinds of excuses and "logical" reasons to explain why you can't improve your lot, and by giving conflicting orders to your Active Mind.

Two exercises will help you become more aware of your Directing Mind at work.

Exercise 1: During the day, listen to your "inner chatter" the interior conversations your Directing Mind has with itself. Be aware of how you make judgments, critiques, and analyses of your own actions and what goes on around you. Notice how often you take a situation that has already occurred and review it mentally over and over, making criticisms, evaluations, and justifications. Think about how much good this does you.

Exercise 2: During the day, be aware of how many times you make pictures in your head of the future. Think of how many of those pictures represent positive events and how many are negative. And think of how often you make decisions about how to act, decisions that are based on the emotions stirred up by those pictures produced by your

Directing Mind. Think about the fact that those mental pictures of the future tend to attract similar experiences when you have repeated them often.

The Active Mind

This is the real workhorse of the trio. Your Active Mind is in charge of all your body functions, the operation of your nervous system, your physical behavior and actions, your senses, the distribution of your energy supply (including your emotions), the broadcasting of your thoughts, the operation of your habits, and your memory. It is often referred to as the Subconscious, but that term leaves a lot to be desired because too many people associate it with an uncontrollable part of yourself that often works against you and hides information from you. It's true that you don't know how it does its work, but you can be aware of why it does what it does, and you will find that it is actually a friend, not an enemy. A somewhat better term than subconscious is Body Mind.

I call it the Active Mind because its most basic function is to carry out orders, to act and react rather than to think in the usual sense of that word. It operates very much like a supercomputer, and it often gets blamed for just doing its duty. On the one hand, it follows the orders encoded in the genetic make-up of your cells; on the other hand, it also tries to follow the orders given by the Directing Mind. It deserves more compassion than censure because sometimes the orders of the Directing Mind conflict with the orders of the cells. This might happen when the Directing Mind decides that overeating is a good substitute for affection. Sometimes, too, the Directing Mind gives orders that conflict with other orders—its own, given previously—as when someone goes ahead and does something he has already decided is morally wrong. In both cases the immediate result is stress and tension, which may lead to illness and/or undesirable circumstances.

Its function as the guardian of habits reaps the most abuse for the Active Mind. You should know by now that all habits originate in conscious decisions made by the Directing Mind that have been reinforced by repeated attention and imagery until the Active Mind obeys them automatically. The fact that the Directing Mind often "forgets" what it did to bring about the habit means that it usually blames the Active Mind (by whatever name) instead of itself for undesirable habits over which it thinks it has no control. The truth is that habits of thought and behavior originated with the Directing Mind, and can be changed by it using the tools previously discussed.

Now, for some ways to get better acquainted with this Active Mind, here are some exercises.

Exercise 1: An excellent suggestion made by a man named Max Long was to give your Active Mind a personal name of its own to make communication and order-giving easier. A great many people have had a lot of success with this. It is something like giving a name to a computer, only in this case the "computer" actually responds in a positive way to such focused attention. So give it a name of your own choosing and use the name when you want better performance from your body, your memory, and your emotions, and when you are using the mental tools to establish new habits. Use the name as well to thank your Active Mind when it does perform like you want. You may be surprised at the response. Long suggested using the name George (from "Let George do it!"), some people use their own middle names, and others pick a name of a favorite character from history or fiction. Use what feels good.

Exercise 2: Being the storehouse for memory is an important function of the Active Mind. Perhaps surprisingly, it seems to have preferences for certain memories over others. The memories that it prefers, and the emotions that may be related to those memories, can give you a lot of information about your own operating ideas and beliefs. One way to tap into these memories is by a process called "treasure-hunting." What you do is find a quiet spot to sit, take a few deep breaths, relax your muscles, close your eyes, and, using the name you've given it, tell your Active Mind to present you with its favorite memories. Then you just wait for them, to rise into awareness. It is important that you refrain from telling it *which* memories to present. For the moment you are not interested in the preferences of your Directing Mind. Just give the order to present the memories it prefers, and wait. You'll know it is working when "treasures" appear that you have probably consciously forgotten. They are likely to be short, vivid, and full of sensory detail. If nothing appears, try again at another time, using one of the Emotivation exercises to relax. Then explain carefully to yourself exactly what you want. Have patience, it will happen.

As with your Creative Mind, the more you "make friends" with your Active Mind, the more positively it will work for you.

Part II

Chapter Seven

The Mirror of Your Body

"The body is a magnificent machine!" This phrase or something similar is what you are likely to hear from an orthodox health practitioner who is impressed with the wonderful way in which the body operates. Well, it *is* magnificent. Quite on its own it takes in oxygen from the air and somehow causes it to enter the bloodstream, while during the same process it expels waste gases. It digests our food, extracting the nutrients, getting rid of what it can't use. It pumps an amazing amount of blood through the circulatory system to feed and cleanse all the cells, and it keeps replacing old cells with new ones. It produces special cells and organs to deal with infection, and others to emit necessary chemicals or transmit sensations. It is indeed magnificent. But it is most decidedly not a machine.

The idea of the body as a machine grew with the development of the Industrial Age, which is still very much with us. It is true that there are many similarities between the body and a machine. Both are made of components with different functions, both do work, both generally have moving parts, and both seem to break down or wear out. Influenced by machine-age thinking, health practitioners began to treat the body as a machine. If something went wrong with it, then there had to be a mechanical cause. It might be a short circuit (a breakdown in the nervous system), a faulty or worn out part, the introduction of something from the outside (germs, bacteria, viruses, poisons) that interfered with its functioning, or the failure on the part of the operator to supply something necessary for its functioning (like vitamins, protein, etc.). All the parts and their various possible difficulties were given labels so that different body mechanics could be sure they were discussing the same thing.

Now it's true that treating the body like a machine has allowed many people to lead longer, productive lives by introducing or replacing chemicals such as drugs and vitamins; by corrective surgery and replacing parts; and by getting rid of parts that were undesirable or no longer functioned well. But it is also true that many lives have been scarred or lost by the same kinds of treatment. Much worse, it has tended to generate an atmosphere of mistrust of one's own body, which might stop working properly at any moment, and a mistrust of the environment, which might attack it at any moment. Even worse than that, the mechanical approach shoved the mind aside, relegating it to the position of a helpless observer except, supposedly, in the case of specialists with inside knowledge.

However, the body is not a machine. For one thing, it always cures itself, sometimes with the help of the "mechanics" and sometimes in spite of them. When a doctor does something to help a body, he is never sure how it is going to react. Maybe it will get well and maybe it won't, but all he can do is hope that what he does will have a good effect. If it doesn't, then he will try something else. If a lot of different *somethings* don't work, he may just give up, but to everyone's surprise the body might get well anyway. Why? Because doctors do not and cannot cure anything, and the best of them will admit it. They can do no better than set up conditions, to the best of their ability, in which a cure might take place. They are usually good at getting rid of specific symptoms, but that's not the same as a cure.

To be accurate, a sick body can't really cure itself either.

The extra, *necessary* factor, is the mind of the individual with the sick body. Getting well, or preventing illness, depends almost entirely on what is going on in that mind. This isn't a new idea by any means. Hippocrates, the "father of modern medicine," among others, subscribed to it. But the idea got buried around the time that machines got popular. Well, not buried exactly; out of favor is more like it. A few health practitioners never completely shoved the mind out of the picture, and more and more are bringing it back in today. This "revolt" within the realms of orthodoxy is known as the field of psychosomatics.

The Psychosomatic Limitation

The word "psychosomatics" was popularized in the 1930s when it was used in a book by Dr. Helen Flanders Dunbar called *Emotions and Bodily Change*. Since then a great deal of important work has been done to show the relationship between mental states and physical health. The result is a clear record of the highly significant role that the mind plays in creating and curing illness. One survey claims that three out of four illnesses have a psychosomatic origin, while another claims that as much as 90% of all lower back pain is psychosomatic. Unfortunately, the field of psychosomatics suffers from several severe limitations.

In the first place, the word itself is practically a misnomer for what is being studied. "Psychosomatics" is based on two Greek words: *Psyche,* meaning *"soul"* or *"mind;"* and *soma,* meaning "body." The implication is that psychosomatics deals with the relationship between ideas and the body. What specialists in the field concern themselves with for the most part, however, is the relationship between emotions and the body, as the title of Dunbar's work indicates. This is certainly better than ignoring the emotions, but it is not yet a true mind/body study. Emotions are energy, and the release of locked up energy can relieve a great deal of pain and suffering, but although symptoms can be thus relieved, no cure will result unless the ideas that generate the emotional blockages are changed. To date, this is still a neglected area.

Another limitation is the connotation or interpretation that the word psychosomatic has been given by many health practitioners and laymen. All too often it is used to mean *imaginary*, in the sense of not being real, as if the person with the symptoms were faking them or were so crazy he didn't know what was happening. Usually this meaning is applied when the doctors or whoever can't find an "organic" cause for the illness (organic here means a visible defect in a body part). Yet "organic" malfunctions of all kinds are merely the end result of malfunctions of thought and emotion, not the cause of illness.

A third limitation is the preoccupation with events as the major cause for mental/emotional states that bring on illness. So-called "stressful events" from childhood, or the recent past, or one's current environment are frequently blamed for illness in the psychosomatic point of view. In childhood it might be the domineering or rejecting parent who is blamed for the stress. Recent studies have shown a strong correlation between events like marriage, death in the family, change of residence or job, breaking off relationships, and similar traumas, and the experience of illness of some kind within twelve months after the event. Correlations are also being made between "stressful" situations such as freeway driving, unpleasant environments at home or work, and economic conditions, and various illnesses. In most of these, the stressful nature of the situation is emphasized. I'd like to point out, though, that this is very much a mechanical approach. In engineering, stress is an outside force applied to an object that may or may not cause it to break down, depending on the amount of force and the strength of resiliency of the object. In the human body, mechanical stress is produced when muscular or cellular tension is in operation, or when an actual physical object or force (i.e., loud sound or bright light) comes in contact with the body. But in and of themselves, *events do not produce stress*. The stress associated with certain events comes from your *reaction* to the event, not the event itself. And that reaction is determined by your beliefs about the event or about yourself in relation to it.

Your Survival System

Built right into your genetic code is a wonderful system for survival that usually goes by the name of "instinct." It's something we share with the animals and it is under the care of our Active Mind. Part of this system has been identified as a "flight or fight" response, and some researchers have noted a link between this response and illness. I want to go farther and show you that you have four survival responses that are directly linked with your state of health or illness. These four responses are Defend, Retreat, Act, and Rest.

Defend: I think this term is more accurate than "fight" because aggressive action does not necessarily involve violence. It could involve something as simple as a frown to indicate your displeasure and a warning to whomever incurred it. Basically, it has to do with asserting yourself to defend whatever you believe is important to your survival (i.e., your food supply, your rights, your integrity, your person). When it does involve violence, it's because you believe violence is necessary, regardless of whether it actually is necessary.

Retreat: Again, I think this is more accurate than the term "flight" because it includes simple responses such as closing your mouth when you see your words are getting you into trouble. Actual flight, ranging from walking away calmly to running full tilt, is only a part of this survival response.

Act: As a survival response, this one has to do with supplying your basic needs like food, sex, exercise, and communication, none of which necessarily involve defending or retreating.

Rest: This simply refers to your basic instinct for sufficient physical rest and sleep.

This survival system is intimately connected to your state of health. When your Directing and Active minds are working in harmony and your instincts are followed appropriately, that is, with due consideration given to your circumstances, then you will be in a state of vibrant health.

But a disruption of the survival system results in ill health.

Such a disruption comes about when your Directing Mind gives contradictory orders in a survival situation. Then, instead of a simple "defend" or "retreat" order, for example, you might be giving "defend/don't defend" or "retreat/don't retreat." At that point your body begins to protest by sending you messages of pain, illness, or malfunction. Please note this well: Pain, illness, or malfunction in your body is not a punishment, it is a message that there is a conflict of ideas that threaten your survival.

Conflicting orders to your survival system produce acute or chronic tension in your muscles or cells until the conflict is resolved. Drugs, food, deep breathing, massage, and other techniques may temporarily reduce or mask the tension, but it will quickly build back up again as long as the conflict exists. That's why your beliefs have so much to do with your health. Now let's look at some examples of typical conflicts.

Defend/Don't Defend: If, as a child, you accepted a belief that it is wrong to assert yourself or to show anger, that by itself might not cause you any physical difficulty. You could simply resort to the Retreat mode of survival and avoid any conflict. But if you also held the belief that asserting yourself is necessary to your survival, then every time you faced a situation in which the Defend instinct was aroused, it would automatically be contradicted by the first belief. The amount of tension resulting would depend on the strength of the emotions aroused by the situation, which the conflict would repress.

Retreat/Don't Retreat: Some people grow up with the idea that the best survival course to follow is to retreat from threatening situations. That might produce a milquetoast personality, but not necessarily ill health. If a male child developed that belief *plus* a belief that a man must always be assertive, then such a conflict in the face of threat would probably cause him physical trouble. Simple stage fright could be one result, because having all the eyes of an audience on you can seem threatening. I heard an actor state in an interview that he regularly got deathly ill before every performance, though he was all right once on stage. This was because his body was getting "retreat/don't retreat" messages. On stage he switched to a set of more harmonious "it's okay to act" beliefs. At their worst "retreat/ don't retreat" conflicts may result in paralysis.

Act/Don't Act: A belief that certain activities are wrong, coupled with a strong desire to carry them out can lead to many kinds of physical illness. With this mode, the most obvious conflicts have to do with sex and affection, but it can include such things as dancing, drinking alcohol, or doing particular kinds of work, depending on the individual's beliefs. "Act/Don't Act" may also translate as "Must Act/ Can't Act." Despair and hopelessness can easily result from such a conflict, and it is interesting to note that psychosomatic researchers have found high correlations between such feelings and cancer patients. By the way, I am against the popular phrase "cancer victim" because there is no such thing. Cancer is a reaction to a conflict in beliefs, and not to any outside agent.

Rest/Don't Rest: The body does need a certain amount of rest each day. Probably not as much as you believe, but it does need some. But when a belief that a certain amount of rest is necessary is contradicted by a belief that rest is dangerous, there is sure to be difficulty. How can anyone believe that rest is dangerous? Well, a person who associates sleep with death and who is afraid of dying might come up with such a conflict. So might a person who believes that life is short and they must constantly be on the go to achieve something or to prove themselves worthy of something. The latter beliefs are so common that people who have them are called "Type A" personalities, and usually suffer from hypertension, high blood pressure, or heart problems.

All illness, I am saying, is caused by inharmonious beliefs that affect one's basic survival system. It is not enough to talk about repressed emotions as being the cause of illness because emotions are always repressed for a reason. Anger, jealousy, resentment, anxiety, guilt, etc., are feelings arising from beliefs. They are effects, not causes. To prevent or heal illness you have to deal with the beliefs underlying the conflict. The resolution of such conflicts often occurs spontaneously, in ways that an individual might not even be fully aware of. When it does, there is a spontaneous cure. But this doesn't happen often enough, so it isn't something we can count on. Fortunately, we have Directing Minds that we can use to do the same thing consciously.

Somography and Illness

I enjoy coining words, so here is one coined on the spot just for this book—*somography*. Just as geography is the study of the earth (*geo* = earth) and its division into regions, somography is the study of the body (*soma*) and its division into regions.

A rather curious thing noted by ancients and moderns interested in mind-body relationships is that beliefs and illnesses are strongly inclined to be associated with particular areas of the body. What's more, these areas or regions seem to be divided mostly on a horizontal basis without regard to muscle and skeletal structures. The study of this phenomenon is what I call somography, because I have never run across any other adequate name for it.

Somographic divisions have been made by other authors, notably Wilhelm Reich in *Character Armor*, but my own research has led me to disagree with some of their conclusions. So naturally I am about to present you with my own classification system which I hope will help you in pinpointing the ideas behind your illnesses.

Region I: Head, shoulders, arms and hands.

Region II: Chest, breasts, lungs, heart, and upper back.

Region III: The abdominal cavity, genito-urinary system and lower back and buttocks.

Region IV: Legs and feet.

The chapters to follow will discuss each of these regions and the ideas and illnesses associated with them.

The Right/Left Split

This is another division, one which obviously exists, but one whose meaning in terms of illness is still speculative. This is the so-called right/left or vertical split of the body. In terms of appearance, it means that the right side of your body often looks different than your left side. Sometimes there is a difference in muscular development of the arms or legs which may or may not be due to tension, and sometimes one breast is larger than the other. The clearest difference, however, is in the face. You can check this out for yourself by placing the edge of a mirror on the middle of someone's face in a frontal photograph. Adjust it so that half the face is reflected in the mirror to look like a full face. Then turn the mirror around and do the same with the other side. The difference may startle you, because it may look like two entirely different people. What you are seeing is the reflection of two aspects of the person's personality.

It is likely that this difference has something to do with the fact that the left side of your brain, which scientists have found to be associated with analytical and verbal skills, more or less controls the right side of your body; and the right side of your brain, associated with artistic and integrating skills, has a greater influence on the left side of your body. In practical terms, though, you could say that the right side of your body is more "masculine-oriented" and the left side more "feminine-oriented," using these words to mean general qualities, not sex differences.

I think that this split is part of our natural heritage due partly to the way our brain works and partly to the fact that we have an equal share of chromosomes from male and female parents. In any case, there is some data that indicates that our illnesses tend to "take sides."

According to this idea, illnesses or physical conditions on the right side tend to be involved with male relationships, including the father, while conditions on the left tend to be involved with female relationships, including the mother. It's an interesting idea, but I emphasize that it is still pretty much speculation. Still, it may be worth taking into account when seeking the source of your ideas behind illness.

Something to Keep in Mind

Although the next few chapters will deal with specific regions and parts of the body, it is well to remember that you can have several idea conflicts going on at the same time, so that any given bout of illness can affect more than one region. In addition, certain beliefs can act as "bridges" between the ideas associated with different regions, which is why a condition such as constipation may also result in a headache. Always be aware that you are a whole person, and not just a conglomeration of parts. With that said, let's look at the parts anyway.

CHAPTER EIGHT

Region I — The Communication Center

The head, neck, shoulders, arms, and hands all form what I call the communication center of the body. This area is the one most involved with the communication of thoughts and feelings. The head is in charge of seeing, hearing, tasting, smelling, speaking, and a myriad of facial expressions; the neck moves the head to indicate agreement or disagreement; a shrug or lift of the shoulders can convey a variety of messages; the arms say things with hugs or gestures; and the hands are used for touching, signaling, and modes of expression such as writing, painting, playing music, and others. Besides communication, however, Region I also concerns our sense of achievement, recognition, and competence. In the light of that, we'll begin our study of why things go wrong here.

The Head

Above all, the head is where we most directly confront our thoughts about ourselves and about others. Primarily for this reason it is where we experience that most common symptom of all, the headache. Headaches come mainly from trying to suppress certain kinds of thoughts because we are afraid to think them. You may fear that the thoughts themselves are harmful or "sinful," or you may be afraid that they will reveal things about yourself that you don't want to be aware of. For instance, migraines are often associated with repressed rage, but that doesn't explain why the rage is repressed. The reason is that the person fears the consequences of thinking such angry thoughts, or believes they shouldn't be thought. Yet the thoughts are there, seeking their natural expression, so the orders given are "think/don't think" and a headache results.

Self-criticism and criticism from others can give rise to headaches when you fight against listening to it because it brings into question your achievements or competence. Criticism directed toward others may do the same, especially if you reinforce it by such habitual statements as "(he, she or it) gives me a headache." If you feel a sense of "pressure" to perform in any sense and rebel against it, that can also give you a headache. Actually, the sense of pressure itself comes from the rebellion, because unless your head is physically stuck in a vise the only pressure is in your reaction.

In later chapters I will be describing general self-healing techniques, but at this point I'd like to mention a couple specifically for headaches that others and myself have found quite useful for relieving the pain. The first is to direct your attention to your hands and imagine them getting warmer, as if you were putting them in hot water. This tends to release the tension by directing blood and emotional energy flow away from the head. The second one is just to imagine your head gently expanding, as if it were becoming free and loose. Both of these techniques work well, but they are only symptom relievers. The cause lies with the conflict in thinking. In cases where there is an actual organic disorder, such as a tumor, the cause still lies with the conflict in thinking. As with all organic disorders, the physical manifestation is the end result of long-term intensive tension. By removing the idea conflict you will allow the natural healing processes of the body to do their work.

I'd like to mention a word about fever, which may or may not accompany a headache or extend beyond the head. This is the result of a lesser degree of tension which restricts, but does not block, the flow of emotional energy. In a way, it is like electrical resistance, the kind that heats your iron or toaster. It occurs when you are "burned up" about something. Again, resolving the mental conflict will allow the fever to dissipate.

The Face

Are you afraid to "face up" to something, or concerned with "losing face?" Then the face could be an area of difficulty for you. Irritation at criticism, lack of recognition, or doubts about competence may also result in a facial blemish of some kind. Adolescents seem to have a lot of problems with facial blemishes, but it has less to do with hormonal changes than the fact that they are then beginning to desire recognition as competent adults. When this desire is frustrated by parents or teachers, the suppressed irritation shows clearly on their faces, and the severity of the problem is equal to the degree of suppression. In my own children, I have noticed that the "breaking out" coincides markedly with the state of their relationships with their teachers, my wife and I, and their girlfriends (I have all boys). When they get what they feel is proper recognition, their faces clear up. What adds to the problem for adolescents, however, is the social belief that "this is the age when facial blemishes naturally occur." An acceptance of that belief will produce blemishes even without suppressions related to others, though probably not as bad.

The Eyes

These most important sensory organs are directly involved with the way we "view" life and ourselves in particular. For instance, if you believe the future holds a lot of danger and you don't want to look at it, you could develop a nearsightedness. And if you believe the present holds the most danger, then farsightedness could result. In such cases, corrective glasses merely reinforce those ideas when they are worn habitually, reinforce your dependence on some physical thing to help you, and may also serve as protective shields from other people. Two nearsighted people I have been working with have both experienced great improvement as a result of an increase in general awareness, their sense of competence, and a strong *desire* for improvement enhanced by healing techniques.

Some eye conditions are related to parental resistance. I know of two cases where an astigmatism in the right eye was related to suppressed feelings against the father (remember the right/left split), and in one case it cleared up as soon as the father died. But there's no need to wait for your father to die. All it takes is a resolution of the mental conflict.

Eyestrain, glaucoma, cataracts, loss of vision—all of these and other eye disorders are caused by tension. In the news recently there has been quite a controversy over the use of marijuana to relieve certain eye conditions. The reason it works is because the herb is a notable relaxant. Sometimes the tension is not a result of conflicts over relationships, but of ideas on how to use the eyes. A telephone operator I helped who was having increasing difficulty in reading the small print to read numbers for customers simply believed that it was necessary to squint and strain in order to read better in poor light. When she learned to take a couple deep breaths and relax her eyes through imagination, she found a great improvement in her ability to see without strain.

The state of your eyes is also influenced, to a considerable extent, by that of your parents. If your parents wore glasses, chances are high that you will, too. The determining factor is not heredity, though, but your acceptance of a belief that you will need glasses just as they do. This might include beliefs that it "runs in the family" (it does — through their heads), that you'll need glasses if you read a lot in poor light (there's no scientific proof of that because it's the straining, not the lighting that affects you), or that you'll need glasses when you reach a certain age.

The last belief given can result in what is known in psychosomatics as the "anniversary syndrome." It may affect any part of the body, but we'll discuss it here. The anniversary syndrome works in two ways. In the first one, you may get a particular symptom at the same age as your parent did. This is because somewhere in your belief system is a firm idea that that symptom is supposed to occur at that age. So when that anniversary rolls around in your life, your Active Mind will automatically produce the tension required to bring on the symptom, thus confirming the belief. It is a credit to human ingenuity and creativity that even this can have a survival purpose. A few days ago my wife received a call from a friend in his sixties who said he had just recovered from a heart attack. He then related that his father had had an identical attack at the same age, but then had gone on to live into his eighties. It is possible that this friend believes that the heart attack is some kind of magical guarantee that he will live longer, too, or that it is a "test" that he had to pass.

The second kind of anniversary syndrome is more like celebrating (not exactly a choice word) the "birthday" of some traumatic event in your own life. If you witnessed something extremely unpleasant in the month of December as a child, you might have made associations with December-type weather or holiday trappings or whatever. And so you might develop eye problems every year at about the same time as the incident is recalled and you struggle not to see it. But people who do this often do not make the connection between the physical condition and the anniversary. If you are subject to an anniversary syndrome of some kind, practice the realization that you do not *have* to follow in your parents' physical footsteps, nor do you *have* to go on celebrating sickness.

Poor eyesight may be related to a poor self-image, an overly humble attitude, or a fear of the consequences of appearing aggressive. Among many animals, to look at another directly in the eye is an aggression signal. This is why members of the dog and cat family will usually look away from your stare. This isn't because your superiority as a human has subdued them. They are merely signaling politely that they don't want to challenge you. Among humans, looking one directly in the eye may be a signal for aggression, assertiveness, or a desire for intimacy. That's why it isn't considered polite to stare. And that's why some people will develop poor eyesight, and possibly add protective glasses, so as not to arouse fear-provoking feelings from others.

The Ears

In many cases, earaches and loss of hearing have do with a resistance to hearing criticism, from your inner elf as well as from others. Earaches in particular respond well to tension-releasing exercises. When earaches have reached the point where infection and swelling is adding to the pressure, then obviously it's a good idea to include physical remedies with the relaxing and belief work. Remembe always that the point is to get well, and not to prove any method by its exclusive use. In this book I am emphasizing the application of Imagineering to health, as I stated in the preface, but I am not insisting that we do away with all other forms of treatment, especially those tha´ involve common sense. This was brought home to me in a signif cant way while helping a woman who was suffering from severe earaches. She told me the doctors had said nothing was wrong physically, so I trained her in relaxation techniques and methods for resolving the idea conflicts, but we only achieved temporary effects. About a year later she came to see me and said that another doctor had finally found and removed a piece of cotton stuffed way up her ear canal, and that now her ear was fine. Now I personally believe that the finding of the cotton coincided with an inner decision on her part to finally resolve the conflict, but someone had to get that cotton out. Along similar lines, I don't hesitate to use preparations for dissolving earwax when a hard lump of it accompanies an earache—*in addition* to Imagineering techniques.

In our culture, loss of hearing is frequently associated with aging. As with failing eyesight and a number of other symptoms, the main cause of this is the social belief that these things are a natural by-product of old age. They are not. There is no natural reason why you should suffer a loss in any of your sense faculties regardless of your age, as long as you maintain healthy beliefs about them.

Dizziness and loss of balance may be related to problems of the inner ear where our sense of balance is regulated. These symptoms are also related to ideas that your life is seriously out of balance or that things are out of control and so confused as to make you dizzy. The physical effects result from trying to suppress those feelings.

The Mouth

The mouth is the most important organ of communication that we have. As babies we use it to take in food from the outside world, to show displeasure by pushing food back out, or by biting, and as a means of experiencing everything from nipples to sand. As we grow older we use it for the marvelous phenomenon of speaking, as well as for spitting, kissing, and perhaps more biting.

With the mouth we can express the whole range of emotions that we feel, so this area can be the center of a lot of repression. All speech impediments other than those attributed to birth defects are rooted in repression of some kind. Stuttering and lisping are outstanding examples, both of which respond well to relaxation therapy and the building up of self-confidence.

From personal experience I know that the lip condition called herpes or cold sore is due to holding back angry words. Until several years ago I had never experienced this, but probably as a result of my studies of illness, my body-mind got the idea that this would be a good way to let me know when I was repressing angry words (previously it had used other ways). As I learned to tune in to this condition I got to the point where I could feel the cold sore beginning to form shortly after suppressing a hot retort. And although the condition generally has a run of three days or more, I have been able to look in the mirror and watch it disappear in as little as an hour by releasing the emotions and changing the idea that gave rise to them. What I have done, you can do, too.

74

In regard to expressing emotions, I want to bring out very forcefully that what I mean by this is allowing yourself to *feel* them freely. In other words, allow yourself full freedom to express them to yourself. You do not have to express them *to* the person you are angry with. The free flow of the emotions is what is important. That means it's not okay to punch the boss in the nose, stomp up and down on your spouse, or swat someone with a brick, but it's still okay to *feel* like doing it. If the feeling is so strong it cries out for physical expression, then scream into a towel, beat a pillow, or stomp on a cardboard box. Use an appropriate outlet that won't get you into trouble, but *feel.* Most, if not all, symptoms could be alleviated to a tremendous degree by following this simple advice. That goes for feelings of anger, fear, jealousy, the whole lot.

Teeth are not only used for eating, they also represent one of our few natural means of defense—biting. We attempt this as a matter of course as children, but we are generally forced to cease and desist as we become able to bite hard enough to hurt. Nevertheless, the urge to bite is still part of our nature, however much we suppress it. For lack of sufficient evidence, I present it as a theory only that tooth decay and other tooth problems are due to the tension resulting from repressing emotions that urge us to bite in the face of mentally perceived or physical danger. Relaxation techniques can relieve a toothache, so tension is involved. It stands to reason, in my mind, that chronic tension might either bring on tooth decay or at least render the teeth more susceptible to outside agents such as sugar. It just might prove fruitful to develop a type of therapy for releasing emotions based on biting and biting motions. I suspect the result would be fewer cavities and better check-ups. I think that in large part the biting urge is a reaction to criticism. The same kind of tension would affect the gums.

The Nose

As the organ of smelling, the nose may play a role in triggering symptoms based on memories of past events that have been associated with particular odors. It is also possible that nose problems can stem from repressed fear of putting your nose in someone else's business. Silly as that might sound, it is typical of the way your Active Mind translates verbal expressions into physical ones. The Active Mind tends to take our habitual verbal expressions literally, so that a fear of being thought "nosy," for instance, could result in symptom-producing tension.

However, as part of the respiratory system, the nose is an important factor in cold symptoms. Although what we call the common cold may involve the eyes, ears, nose, sinuses, throat, and chest, we'll discuss this unpleasant symptom in the present section.

First of all, a cold has little if anything to do with viruses or contagious "bugs." So you won't *catch* a cold from someone else unless you are mentally and emotionally predisposed to do so. Such a predisposition might include being in a similar emotional state, or believing that contact will give you a cold. Believing that drafts, wet feet, cold weather, or getting rain-soaked will cause colds may also bring them on. In and of themselves, all they cause is discomfort. Yet, I venture to say that most cold symptoms are substitutes for, or repressions of, the simple act of crying.

Think about the similarity of the effects: Runny or stuffed up nose, clogged sinuses, watery eyes, choked up throat, sobbing/coughing chest. Crying is often a natural response to feelings of helplessness and frustration. When this natural response is suppressed because of ideas like "men don't cry," "crying is a sign of weakness and I refuse to be weak," and the like, then the ideal conditions are set up for a cold. Now cold symptoms may be relieved by a good cry, but an even quicker method is to acknowledge the feeling of helplessness and frustration, recognize the ideas behind them, and change them. When done thoroughly, this can get rid of cold symptoms in minutes. In my family, where everyone is taught that there is always positive action that can be taken in any situation, no one has had a cold in years. Nevertheless, it ought to be noted that apart from beliefs in how colds are caused and suppressed feelings of frustration, a cold may serve the practical purpose of providing an opportunity for a rest from one's work or relationships. In that case, the best course may be to just live through it, although the suffering is unnecessary.

Other nose conditions that may be related to suppressed crying are frequent sneezing, post-nasal drip (crying backwards), chronic sinus congestion, and spontaneous nosebleeds.

The Throat

The connection of the throat to crying has been mentioned, but it is also the channel by which we accept food into our system. Symbolically (for the Directing Mind, but literally for the Active mind), we tend to associate food with ideas, as evidenced by such expressions as "food for thought," "Do you expect me to swallow that?", "you're feeding me a bunch of baloney," "that idea is unpalatable," and "he was force-fed with the wrong ideas." The throat, then, and the glands and organs in and around it, can swell up and get sore as a repressed response to ideas that are unacceptable. The repression comes from being afraid or believing it is wrong to express such non-acceptance vocally.

In the reverse direction, throat problems may also be a response to stifling response. Out of the throat come the sounds of speech, passion and suffering, and when these well up the throat can swell up if they are cut off with a "don't act" order. A young man I worked with had a throat constriction so severe that hospitalization was recommended. The diagnosis was that it was the result of a physical trauma experienced a week before when a friend had angrily grabbed him by the throat during an argument. I found out from the boy that he had not even rebuked the friend, but had simply kept silent about it. Before taking the step of hospitalization I helped him for a couple of hours with relaxation techniques and by encouraging him to express his feelings about the incident, assuring him that it was not unmanly to do so. During that time he did release his feelings, expressing his deep hurt with great sobs while I gave him support. Afterwards he slept all night and in the morning he was perfectly well. If those two hours hadn't helped, I would have sent him to the hospital with my blessing, but in this case it was fortunately not necessary.

Tonsilitis and swelling of the lymph and salivary glands in the throat may also be due to similar repression. The first time I ever got tonsilitis was in the Marine Corps on a training exercise when I felt I was unjustly reprimanded and wasn't allowed to defend myself (my competence was questioned). At that time I was treated by antibiotics, but I successfully used imagineering techniques on a couple of later flare-ups. But antibiotics can be very helpful in treating tonsilitis or strep throat, so don't disdain them or refuse out of hand. Always use what works, though you will usually find that medicines work better when combined with imagineering.

The Neck

Here I'll just say a few words regarding stiffness and pain.

As a child I was rather "stiff-necked," a stubborn tyke who didn't like to yield to opinions I thought were wrong. And so I often suffered from a stiff neck. One occasion that stands out in my memory is when I was sent to a California grade school, at my mother's insistence, all dressed up in a suit and tie. Needless to say it was grossly inappropriate, and needless to say the stiffness was centered on the left side of my neck. Today I am no less stubborn, but I'm not afraid to express it.

A pain in the neck can not only be a pain in the neck, but also a reaction to a person or situation that is a pain in the neck. Such pain is invariably due to tension, often aggravated or brought on by frequent statements or thoughts to the effect that the person or situation is what you're feeling. My wife used to get neck pains whenever she had to drive on a crowded freeway. She could have successfully imagineered her way out of that by changing her attitude toward crowded freeways, but she chose an equally successful alternative: She avoids them.

The Shoulders

The shoulders are an amazingly expressive part of your anatomy. A simple shrug can say, "Who knows?", "What can I do about it?" or "So what?" A slight turn of the shoulder can signal someone that they are not welcome in your company. And one rotating shoulder on a pretty lady can signify an exaggerated intimate welcome. The shoulders may also be a mirror of our habitual feelings and beliefs about life. "Square" shoulders exude an attitude of confidence in one's ability to deal with anything. High, straight shoulders show that one is in a chronic state of fear, as if he were expecting to be hit from behind at any moment. Overly sloped shoulders give the impression that one believes life is too great a burden to bear. Shoulders that are hunched forward like a prizefighter's reveal that one is in a constant state of readiness for attack. A relative of mine has shoulders that are dramatically hunched and sloped, indicating that, in his view, life is a tough struggle. Shoulders that are always pulled way back seem to be showing that one is making a great effort not to attack. Curiously, this is often accompanied by an aggressively out-thrusting chin, as if inviting someone else to take the first poke.

A surprising number of people do not have real freedom of movement with their shoulders. While teaching classes on a Polynesian form of "meditation in movement" called *Kalana,* I noticed that a majority of students had great difficulty in moving their arms freely away from their body. It was as if they felt a habitual need to keep their arms protectively close. In looking at people in general, it seems to be a prevalent habit and that's an obvious sign that there are a lot of fearful people about. It's chronic shoulder tension that inhibits the free swinging of the arms. The more confident you are, the more at ease you will be with wide arm movements.

From the shoulders, we move our arms to reach out to people and things, to hug with affection, and to hit in anger. When the emotional force of these impulses is counter-manded, the result can be severe inhibition of movement, pain, and/or bursitis. Relaxation techniques can do wonders, but proper work with the ideas in conflict can keep it from happening again.

The Arms

Problems with the arms hinge primarily on the elbow. As with all joints, stiffness, or swelling there may be a product of inflexible thinking. At the elbow, it is likely to be involved with resistance in the area of achievement or your sense of competence. There might also be resistance to being "elbowed out" of some situation, or a conflict about "elbowing your way in." You might even be reluctant to use "elbow grease" on some situation that you know needs work.

The arms themselves are mostly subject to skin irritations like rashes, itching, boils, etc. Ask yourself whether someone or something is irritating you, if you think you are being too rash about something, if you are itching to hit someone or accomplish something but feel frustrated, or whether you are boiling inside. Skin conditions anywhere on the body may occur when inner conflicts are surfacing. On the arms it will have to do primarily with ideas related to competence, recognition, and achievement.

The Hands

These fantastic appendages have an incredible range of expression and utility. They can actually speak our thoughts through literature, art, music, sign language, and gestures. A number of years ago I saw a play in which a man and a woman met, fell in love, were tragically separated, and later joyfully reunited. The remarkable thing is that it was done without words or props, and the main characters were a pair of hands.

Hands may be used to build or destroy, to caress or punch, to give or grab, to hold on or let go, to explore or push away. In their form and lines they can offer clues to age, sex, personality, and career. Because of their amazing versatility they are subject to a wide variety of mental conflicts, all of which essentially center around communication and accomplishment.

Poor circulation resulting in chronically cold hands may be related to a conflict between a desire and a fear of reaching out to touch someone. Sweaty hands are more likely due to a fear of making mistakes or appearing foolish (incompetent). Cramps or other difficulties might arise from resistance to "giving someone a hand" or to receiving handouts. Or there could be a conflict about being able to "handle" things. I know a woman who injured both thumbs shortly after wondering to herself why she was losing her grip on things.

People who use their hands extensively in their work, like writers, musicians, and artists, may suffer extreme cramps when they are in conflict about their ability or what they are communicating. I read of a case where a man who thought of himself primarily as an artist got a bad cramp while writing due to guilt over not using his "normal" means of expression *and* over a sense of not being able to communicate verbally with his mother.

Arthritis, a painful inflammation of the joints, is a very common hand affliction. It has been found that the typical arthritic has a more or less rigid, perfectionistic, and controlling personality (though the control might be exercised very subtly). Here we have inflexibility, severe self-criticism and criticism of others repressed and mirrored in the hands. Relaxation techniques are very helpful on a temporary basis, but a change of attitude can get rid of the condition altogether. I have witnessed a remarkable transformation in the hands of a woman who began affirming her own competence and worth, along with the use of relaxation methods.

Along with everything else, the hands have a tremendous potential for emitting healing energy. Some of the ways to do this will be given in Part III.

CHAPTER NINE

REGION II — THE IDENTITY CENTER

The Chest

The chest area of the body, including the region between the diaphragm and the neck, is where we subconsciously place our identity. I know most of us think of our "mind" as being in our head if we think about it at all, but our spontaneous sense of identity is a little further down. If you've ever seen an old Tarzan movie you may remember the hero coming up and saying "Me Tarzan" as he pounds his chest. That wasn't because he was brought up by gorillas. It's the most natural human thing in the world to touch or point to your chest when emphasizing that "I" am expressing an opinion or "I" have a certain amount of importance or "I" am feeling particularly happy (the latter often with both hands). This kind of identity gesture crosses all cultural barriers. It would be just as easy to point to your head, but we don't. It's as if, on a biological level, our identity is inside our chest. It turns out that the same is true on the emotional and belief levels, too.

Since this is an identity center, it is where our body harbors ideas relating to self-worth, rejection, compassion (identification with others), and assertiveness, pride, or humility. In its broadest meaning, you can include integrity, one's sense of continuity as a whole being. The feelings most commonly associated with this area are joy (which a great many people call love), and fear (either of a loss or for one's life). The former type is usually quite emotionally sensitive, while the latter is quite insensitive, or at least tries to be. It is no accident that "good military posture" requires a puffed up chest, because among professional soldiers insensitivity is a virtue.

The Breasts

One of the most abominable statements I have ever heard was expressed by a surgeon a year or so ago. He had the idea that all baby girls should have mini-mastectomies right after birth so that there would be no danger of breast cancer when they grew up. This is an extreme example of where machine-type logic can take you. The body is a machine, ergo, make adjustments in the machine before anything goes wrong. What's so scary is that he was so serious.

Breast cancer occurs primarily with women, and it is a direct effect of conflicts about their self-worth. It is intimately tied in with the repression of feelings having to do with an extreme fear of rejection. Such women typically have great difficulty in expressing emotions because not only are they afraid of the feelings, they are afraid of the ideas behind the feelings. One of the principal ideas is "I am so unworthy that no one would accept me if they really knew me." But if they completely believed in their unworthiness they would have less of a problem. The thing is, in our society women are both glorified and disdained. And one effect of this can be the "I am unworthy/I am worthy" conflict. Supporting the positive side is a deep biological and spiritual knowing that one is worthy simply because one exists. The negative side is enhanced by many things, among which are religious concepts that deny individual worth, and the worth of women in particular. As one example, it seems obvious that years of pounding one's breast and saying "Lord, I am not worthy" or "Lord, I am a worthless sinner" is going to have *some* effects on what one believes about oneself. While not every woman with breast cancer may be subject to this particular conditioning, the same kinds of beliefs have taken hold.

Cancer is a disease of extreme chronic tension, the end result of long conflict. In a way it is like self-rejection, because almost always there is a great sense of guilt involved. Along with the guilt is a great feeling of hopelessness, frustration, and a sense of inadequacy in controlling various aspects of life. Now, what is it that we really can't control in life? Other people's behavior (it can be influenced, but not controlled), past events, and future happenings. Cancer patients typically believe that the world is such a dangerous place that it must be controlled, yet they don't believe they can do it. Still, they have to try because they believe it is necessary for the sake of survival. So the body conflict becomes "I must control — I can't control." Such control usually includes attempts to control one's own emotions, too, for "out of control" emotions are not only frightening, they make one feel weak and vulnerable. In a dangerous world, that can be extremely threatening. Cancer is cured, not when a piece is taken out of the body or destroyed by chemicals or radiation, but when one either ceases to believe in the necessity for personal control or becomes convinced that one can effectively cope. When the sense of threat is not so extreme, benign tumors can occur instead of cancer.

The Lungs

Breath is almost a universal symbol for life, and the lungs are the center of our desires and yearnings to experience more of life, to expand ourselves, and to share life with others. Therefore, they are also the center of our fears about such things.

Asthmatics generally have a number of fears related to the above. This I know from personal experience, because I had bronchial asthma as a child. I "grew out" of those symptoms, but years later, during a weekend seminar designed to put one in touch with areas of emotional conflict, I had a tremendous experience of release in the chest area. Along with great sobbing, I felt and expressed an incredible sense of "being okay" (self-worth) and a surge of love for everyone. What had happened was a resolution of conflicts that had kept me from fully expressing those feelings all the time. Since then, on an experimental basis, I have been able to partially induce the old childhood symptoms by reliving my childhood ideas. As soon as I changed the ideas, the symptoms went away.

Below are some of the typical conflicts that an asthmatic may experience:

— a need for dependence (usually starting with a parent) and a desire for independence;
— being out of harmony with the environment;
— a desire for and a fear of being assertive (the fear is because others might oppose or reject);
— fear of not doing what others want or expect and resentment at being manipulated;
— guilt from not living up to expectations;
— loss of a loved one or rejection by others.

Asthmatics also have a tendency to experience the anniversary syndrome. When the conflicts are not so severe, the result may simply be a non-specific "ache" in the chest.

Smoking certainly pollutes the lungs, but I am convinced that of itself it does not cause cancer. That is the result of emotional conflicts similar to those already discussed. Because shallow breathing is often a defense against experiencing feelings of fear, I think smoking can be a sort of unconscious compensation to provide an opportunity for deeper breathing. Deep breathing also induces relaxation, so smokers trying to kick the habit may get irritable and tense because they are reverting to defensive shallow breathing. When the fear conflicts are resolved, the habitual need for smoking will diminish or disappear. That's why some people can quit overnight and others go through agony, perhaps partly as a form of self-punishment and justification. I recognize, of course, that smoking may also be tied in with a felt need to keep the hands occupied, oral pleasure, and the comfort of familiar ritual as well as peer pressure.

As a final comment on lung cancer, someone very close to me died with it, and shortly after I was amazed to read in a book on psychosomatics that a person with lung cancer typically has experienced the loss of a parent before the age of fifteen, marital problems, and professional frustration. This person had all those things, and I know he died of hopelessness, not cancer. Now, cancer doesn't automatically occur if those conditions are present, but they do provide a framework in which hopelessness can take hold.

The Heart And Blood System

In literature, speech, and song, the heart is associated with feelings of love, compassion, grief, rejection, yearning, and belonging, and fear. You "give your heart" to someone you love (or leave it in places like San Francisco), and you experience "heartache" or "heartbreak" if that love isn't returned. If compassionate, you are "bighearted," and if not, you might have "no heart" or be called "hard-hearted" or "cold-hearted." A great loss might "break your heart" and you may give "heartfelt thanks" to someone else who is compassionate. In fear, your heart might skip a beat or find its way mysteriously into your mouth. All of these feelings have their biological reflections.

The heart is a muscle, and as such it is subject to acute or chronic tension. People with heart problems tend to be those who are trying to block feelings of compassion or rejection. Compassion could be blocked because it might be interpreted as a sign of weakness, especially by a person who believes in a dangerous world, and that one must be ruthless (without compassion) to get ahead. Probably more common is the person who suppresses fears of rejection and desperately tries to buy love or acceptance through personal achievement or the accumulation of money and material goods. Such a person is often described as "Type A" personality, typified by a driving need to justify their worth in some material way, because otherwise they would feel worthless — unworthy of love. Telling this person to relax and take it easy does little good until they begin to believe that they don't need to prove their worth by what they do to please others. Too many times a person like this will get so involved in the proving that they end up ignoring, and thus losing, the love of the very ones they think they are doing it for. And sometimes they are trying to buy the love of parents either long gone or who refuse to be impressed by anything. What is required for most heart patients is a whole new view of life, in which beliefs in rejection are rooted out and replaced by true self-esteem.

The blood system is naturally linked to the heart, and subject to such conditions as hypertension, anemia, and leukemia. What these three have in common is that they are associated with beliefs in weakness, incompetence, and helplessness, plus a lot of anger at being treated that way. Self-directed anger at not being able to control things better also may be included. These people are usually very manipulative and very resentful at being manipulated. Leukemia in particular often appears shortly after a significant loss of a parent or career position, accompanied by intense feelings of frustration from not being able to do anything about it. People with these conditions generally are unable to express their emotions easily. If they could, it would ease the tension considerably.

The Upper Back

If the chest is where we usually experience rejection from others, the back is where we often give it out. This happens, for instance, when you "turn your back" on someone . Symptoms can arise in this area when you are in conflict about "backing down" in response to someone else's aggressiveness, when you're "holding something back" that you feel really ought to be made known, or when you are "holding back" your support or help. Perhaps, most frequently, symptoms occur in this area when you are feeling unduly harrassed and want someone to "get off your back." The back of a young man whom I know felt that way was a mass of red welts and pimples until he left home to strike out on his own. Mind you, it isn't the harrassment that does it, but the refusal to express the feelings about being har-

rassed. And, of course, the belief that one is being harrassed.

The Diaphragm

The diaphragm is a partition or sheet of muscles and ten-
dons that separates the chest cavity from the abdomen. Its
normal function is to help you breathe, but many people
use it to inhibit breathing and feelings of fear, some of
which may be trying to flow up from areas further down.
When this happens the diaphragm becomes tight as a
drumhead, sometimes to the point where a person completely forgets how to breathe deeply.

In the cycle of breathing freely and deeply, it is perfectly
natural for the upper part of the stomach to protrude slightly in part of that cycle. This is only possible when the
diaphragm is allowed to relax. If the diaphragm is
chronically tight then you can't breathe to your full capaci-
ty. Biologically, this reduces your oxygen supply. Emotionally, it keeps you from experiencing uncomfortable
feelings. Mentally, it represents an attempt at self-control.
People I've worked with who consciously induce deep
breathing to the point of relaxing diaphragm tension report
that at first there is a fearful sense of "falling apart" and
then a flood of emotions and memories that seem over-
whelming. After that passes, they say they feel "cleansed,"
like after a good cry.

There are many different kinds of techniques for releasing diaphragm tension, but the best one I've come across is
laughter. A good, hearty dose of laughter will shake up your
system and release an awful lot of built-up tension. It's
been called the "best medicine," and for very good reason.
It will cleanse your system even better than crying or drugs.
And of all the things to laugh about, we ourselves are the
funniest.

CHAPTER TEN

Region III — The Security Center

In this region I'm including the abdomen, the pelvis, and the lower back. It is a region of primary, instinctual drives all related in some way to your sense of security, of being nurtured, and of sharing your physical world with others. It touches on affection and the lack of it, as well as possessiveness and support.

The Stomach

This is the principal area dealing with your instinctual hunger drive. The stomach receives and digests your food, and when it gets too empty it hurts as a message to get you to do something about it. The intake of food is one of the very first pleasures you experience in this world, and the filling of the belly produces a sense of relaxation, comfort, and security. But, as I've mentioned previously, food represents other things besides nutrition.

Because you are dependent on others for your first food supply, its effect on the stomach gets associated with how much others care about you. That caring becomes equivalent to survival, or security, because you have to have food to live. And so it becomes truly possible to "hunger" for affection. When this happens to people who believe they do not, or can't, get enough affection to satisfy them, they generally take one of two courses of action. One course consists of substituting food for affection, and this happens to be a very common part of obesity. The obsession with sweets which many fat people have is because in the language of food, sweetness equals affection even more than other kinds of food. People who crave sweets crave affection, it's as simple as that. Because the overeating is a substitute, the real feeling is suppressed and such people often refuse to admit to themselves or others what they really want. The second course is to "unconsciously" shrink the stomach so that less food/affection is required, which can lead one to becoming excessively thin. This is an attempt to refute the need so that one's security sense is less threatened, but it is still a tension situation.

Food

Food represents material security, too, which is why career conflicts and the lack of job satisfaction are frequently involved in stomach troubles. Witness the phrase "He hasn't got the stomach for that kind of work." When job or financial security is "eating away" at someone, it may eat away at the stomach lining in the form of an ulcer. Stomach problems can flare up over fear of the loss of possessions, also. Of course, if you think of certain people in your life as belonging to you, then any threatened loss of their presence could upset your stomach. The feelings associated with this potential loss are what we call jealousy, though that can be tied in with rejection fears as well. Envy, the feeling that you ought to have what someone else has, can upset your stomach, too.

And food represents ideas, which is why we have such sayings as "I've no stomach for his opinions," "That's a disgusting thought," and "I'm having trouble digesting what you said." It's nauseating to think what we can do to ourselves sometimes, isn't it?

The Gall Bladder

The function of this organ is to receive a bitter substance called bile from the liver and transfer it into the small intestine to help break down fats in our food. The emotional components have to do with additional meanings of "gall" and "bile." We speak of an exceptionally irritating person, or one who is outrageously forward as having "a lot of gall," and bile has very old associations with bitterness and anger. When such feelings of bitterness toward another person are allowed to repressively accumulate, they can harden into a gallstone, which is a very painful way for your body to tell you to change your mode of thinking.

The Intestines

These organs complete the digestive process and prepare waste products for expulsion. They act as a holding area, and this is how they are most often translated emotionally. You may have heard of small children who hold back their bowel movements as a means of frustrating their mothers. Well, adults do the same thing as a means of trying to hold on to situations or people. The result is either chronic constipation or intestinal ulcers or some other disorder. They can't really control the outer situation, so they try to control a substitute. When they learn to "let go" then the body functions normally again.

The intestines are the repository for a lot of feelings regarding affection and security, too. What we see as a "pot belly" is not so much the stomach as enlarged intestines in people who have difficulty expressing their real hungers. Intestinal hernias result from tension conflicts about the same ideas. These instinctual feelings are often called "gut knowledge."

Irritation of the rectum and hemorrhoids come from holding on too tightly to things and people that seem to be slipping away. Diarrhea is more a case of desperately trying to get rid of what you don't like, or running away from a situation. I think that was surely the case when we all had the "runs" in boot camp. And I strongly suspect that when this condition appears among tourists far from home in a strange land, it really reflects a semi-conscious dislike of their current surroundings. In all my seven years of traveling through the African bush country, I never had a single case of diarrhea. I loved that adventure. When I did get it, it was on coming back to the city to work in my office again.

The appendix is a finger-like extension of the intestine which traps poisons. Based on work I've done with several people who have had appendicitis, I'm of the opinion that, like gallstones, it occurs after a long period of repressing bitterness toward someone or something. At least one woman was able to make a definite connection between her appendicitis attack and two years of harboring very bitter feelings toward a certain man.

The Liver

The liver has the function of storing sugar, making bile and filtering some poisons out of the blood. It can also be the storehouse for a lot of repressed anger related to thwarted affection and self-dislike. "High livers" — those who gorge themselves on rich foods and alcohol to mask their frustrations — often have bad livers.

Excessive drinking of alcoholic beverages has a seriously detrimental effect on the liver and it plays a part in a complex emotional syndrome. People do not drink to excess because they have developed an addiction to alcohol itself. They do it because the alcohol provides something they believe they need to survive. It provides a temporary release from unbearable tension because of its relaxation effect; it provides an affection substitute because alcohol is changed into sugar in the body; and it provides a numbness that helps to protect one against feelings one is afraid to feel. The liver becomes damaged not only because it can't handle the toxic overload, but because it, too, is subject to the emotional tensions that give rise to the craving for alcohol's benefits. It is commonly thought that alcoholism cannot be cured because it is a physical addiction, and that the only solution is complete abstinence. However, there is a doctor in California who claims to cure alcoholics by helping them to change the beliefs that gave rise to emotional conflicts underlying the problem. I have heard two of his former patients discuss this cure and both said they no longer have any need for alcohol, but they take an occasional drink if they feel like it. Once the conflict is resolved, the need for excessive alcohol to mask the conflict disappears. Alcoholism can be cured because it is an emotional addiction, not a physical one. The key is a willingness and a desire to change beliefs that cause repressed anger and resentment.

Compulsive overeating leading to obesity is strikingly similar to alcoholism in its effects and causes. The liver is again affected because it gets overloaded and is a tension center. As mentioned, food acts as a relaxant, helping to relieve tension temporarily, and serves as an affection substitute. The fat can serve several purposes. For one thing, it acts as a sort of "security blanket" to guard against material/emotional lack. It is also stored energy — emotional energy that is usually based on a great deal of anger and resentment. This energy may take the form of fear, in which case the fat acts like a "buffer," a kind of armor that keeps people at a distance even while the person craves closeness. And in some cases it is used to increase one's importance and presence, a symbol of power and the desire to "throw one's weight around."

The Kidneys/Bladder

This pair of organs, each one capped by an adrenal gland, is concerned with filtering the blood and converting waste products into urine. In Oriental medicine, the kidneys, as well as the adrenals, are considered to be directly linked to the sexual function. I tend to agree with that link since urine is discharged through the sex organs and the body consciousness does relate to itself in terms of similarity of function. This means that kidney troubles are probably closely associated with emotional conflicts related to sex. Although this is still speculative, you can be sure that the emotional repressions typical of Region III are involved. Based on the cases of people with whom I have worked, I am more certain that the bladder, where urine from the kidneys is stored, is related to ideas about sex, and that often bladder infections are due to tension resulting from repression of sexual feelings.

The Pancreas/Spleen

These two organs secrete hormones that modify the composition of the blood, particularly the sugar/insulin levels. The repression involved is usually intense anger in response to loss or threatened loss of affection and security. The typical diabetic, for instance, is a very angry person who is so afraid of that anger that he masks it with apparent docility and helplessness. Not surprisingly, he also has a craving for food (which we know is an affection substitute), and often harbors deep resentment against his parents for not giving him as much affection as he craves. Hypoglycemia, a condition which is sometimes called the opposite of diabetes, may result from similar repressions and conflicts that are simply expressed in a different way. The spleen has long been associated with anger, and "to vent your spleen" is much better than holding it in.

The Lower Back

Did you ever "bend over backwards" to be nice to someone who didn't appreciate it? If so, you may also have developed lower back pain. The pain that occurs here is most often due to "holding back" resentment at someone who is threatening your security or means of support. It can also develop as an unconscious attempt to "back away" from something you don't want to do. I developed a severe lower back pain once that kept me immobile for hours and, "coincidentally" made me lose my job of throwing sacks of cement onto a truck. At the time I didn't make the connection, but I was sure glad not to have to return to work. Far better than drugs for this condition are massage, heat applications, relaxation meditations and, especially, reconciliation of the conflict.

The Sex Organs

As you might suspect, problems with the sex organs or the sexual function are related to fears, guilts, and resentments having to do with sex and sexual relationships. This is fairly obvious with such conditions as impotence and frigidity, but I recommend adding conditions like prostate trouble and venereal disease, too. Conflicting ideas are behind all illnesses. Without the conflict, there is no disease. With the ideas about sex that are rampant in this society it is a wonder that veneral disease isn't even more widespread than it is. It must be because we all unconsciously choose our own means of expressing conflict for our own reasons.

It isn't just conflicts about pure sexual hunger that bring on problems in this area, however. That is an instinctual hunger, but so is the hunger for affection, security, sharing, possessing — and power. In our society sex can be symbolic of any of these, and so sexual difficulties can arise from their related repressions. Some people are so "creative," though, that they can use a sexual dysfunction as a means of exerting power over another.

A striking case that comes to mind is that of a man who became sterile (his body did not produce any live sperm), *only* on those days of the month during which his wife could conceive. He certainly didn't do this consciously. What he did consciously was to repress a deep resentment against her and a desire to get back at her in some way. He wouldn't express it, but the feeling was so intense that his body obeyed in the best way it knew how.

Impotence and frigidity, when not due to fears of sex, are more obvious examples of this kind of power play. Nevertheless, it is repression and tension that brings them about, and that is never healthy.

As laughter is the best tension reliever for Region II, so an orgasm is best for Region III. Unfortunately, many people don't experience this beneficial release to its fullest because of various ideas based on fear. Women may have no orgasms at all or have them rarely, and men may have no more than an ejaculation that barely rates as an orgasm.

A full orgasm not only feels good, but it involves involuntary muscular convulsions that are part of the tension-releasing process. Aside from fears of sex being bad and fears of the opposite sex, the most common reason I've come across in both men and women for incomplete orgasms or none at all is a fear of losing control over oneself. This is tied to ideas about security and trust, and to beliefs that too much pleasure or an abandonment of self-control will lead to self-destruction. Yet, these are only ideas *about* reality, not reality itself. Your body was exquisitely designed to experience an immense amount of pleasure through natural tension-relieving systems like laughter and orgasm. You can establish beliefs that will allow you to take full advantage of these health-giving processes.

CHAPTER ELEVEN

REGION IV — THE PROGRESS CENTER

The legs and feet, which make up this region, reflect feelings and ideas about our position, status, or standing in life; our sense of self-sufficiency; and our reactions to progress, change, and uncertainty.

The Thighs

In spite of the title of this section, some of what follows will necessarily be applicable to the legs in general.

A few years ago I was approached by a woman in a wheelchair who wanted to see if my techniques could do anything for her. Her legs had been completely paralyzed since the age of thirteen (she was in her forties) and she hadn't had any feeling in them for years. She told me that doctors said there was nothing physically wrong, i.e., it wasn't a case of disease or deterioration.

I began by having her do some Imagineering exercises and within three weeks she was delighted and amazed to experience warm currents through her legs. Telling her to keep up the exercises, I then began working on the ideas behind the paralysis. The condition first occurred when she ran home from school after an emotionally traumatic incident involving other students. On arriving home her legs became paralyzed and she hadn't been able to move them since. Although she was reluctant to give details, it was revealed that she had been exceptionally tall for her age. She began to see that the paralysis could have been a kind of drastic solution to "standing out" from the crowd (a very unpleasant experience at thirteen) and perhaps being the butt of jokes and other teenage cruelties. Permanently seated, she was no longer a tall "freak' and could enjoy sympathy in addition.

By working with beliefs and energy flow, more and more feeling came into her legs and it became apparent that there was a real possibility that she might be able to stand up and walk again. At this point, however, she stopped the treatment and I never saw her again. Obviously, the prospect of coping with being tall again was more than she could stand. Not only was there a fear of that, but it was also threatening to her current status as an important officer in an organization for the handicapped where she had many friends. In terms of her own survival beliefs, she made the best choice. This shows that if you want to make a change, you have to want the effects of the change more than you want the *comfort of familiar pain* or inconvenience.

Another woman came to me with a case of partial paralysis. Her condition was a dragging leg due to a lack of free movement at the hip joint. Medication hadn't helped and surgery was not recommended, so I worked with her by inducing energy flow and examining her connected beliefs. The energy techniques were only partly successful. After a good flow stimulation she was able to walk across the room with no trouble, but the condition would soon reappear. Once she went to a healer who specialized in very strong energy flows and after his treatment she was able to walk fine for two days before the condition returned. Her condition was clearly linked to a high degree of tension which the energy flow could only release temporarily because the idea behind it hadn't been touched. It wasn't hard to discover that idea. The condition had started when she had to make a change of residence against her will. Her continued resistance to the change was reflected in her "dragging her feet" (or foot, in this case). Unfortunately, even after that realization she refused to accept the change and so her condition remained. When and if she does accept it she will get better without any help.

You have heard the expression "paralyzed with fear." When the fear is chronic, the paralysis will be reflected in the body. Basically, it's a survival process. Where there is imminent physical danger, temporary paralysis may cause you to be unnoticed and thus save your life. It has worked in certain cases where people have been confronted by bears and lions, and we see such animals as rabbits and opossums use it regularly. Humans may also use it to avoid a situation they don't like or are afraid of, they may experience it when afraid of making a choice between two alternatives, or it may result from resistance to change itself.

Fat may or may not accumulate on the thighs when there is fat elsewhere. If the hips and the thighs are fat, there may be some tie-in with sexual/affectional feelings, but it might be useful to explore beliefs that one is being frustrated from moving forward, especially in a career situation. I have come across such beliefs many times, particularly with women.

The Knees

As a teenager about to go into high school, I became afflicted with a very painful swelling just below the kneecap on both legs. The local doctor in the small town where I lived then diagnosed it as cancer, and for many weeks I went into his office regularly for X-ray treatments. The main effects of the condition were that I had great difficulty in bending my knees, and it seemed that I was constantly bumping into things and yowling with pain. Finally, I was taken to a specialist in a large city hospital who just "happened" to have had the same condition as a child and diagnosed it immediately as something called "Osgood-Schlatter's bone condition." Fairly rare, it was assumed to be due to unusually rapid growth, and he prescribed plenty of milk, lots of rest and the wearing of support bandages. The condition improved only gradually, and it was several years before the tenderness was completely gone.

At the time, of course, it was just something I had to live with, but years later I was able to explore the beliefs behind it. Simply put, it was an extreme result of my not wanting to submit (symbolized by bending my knees), to what I believed was my father's tyrannical nature. At the same time, I felt guilty about feeling that way, so I punished myself by bumping the sore spots at every opportunity. Today I am convinced of two things — that my father was not so tyrannical, and that if I hadn't been so stubborn and inflexible I wouldn't have gotten the condition in the first place.

The knees, then, reflect our feelings about humility, submitting to authority, flexibility regarding status, and fears related to maintaining our position and "standing up" to uncertainties and possible dangers. I recall that in the Marine Corps while forced to stand at attention for hours, quite a few men would keel over as a result of rigidly locking their knees and tensing their leg muscles so as to cut off blood to the brain. Needless to say, they were "scared stiff" of what might happen if they relaxed for an instant. And you know that certain kinds of fear can literally make your knees shake.

The Lower Legs

The lower legs probably get the greatest workout when we are running or walking, so it is not surprising that they often reflect our feelings about moving forward in our career, "climbing the social ladder" or running away from unpleasant situations. Some people who are overly concerned about such things may have beautifully developed calves that look like they exercise a lot, when all they do is sit at a desk or in front of a TV. This is due to frequent unconscious "get moving" signals that keep the muscles working even at rest.

Perhaps the most common condition that can arise in this area is varicose veins, though they can appear elsewhere, too. The symptoms are swollen legs, cramps, fatigue, or pain after long periods of standing, and rather unsightly knots of widened veins just under the skin. The veins, which have the duty of bringing blood back to the heart, contain little valves that are supposed to keep the blood from flowing back down because of the natural pull of gravity. In some people, however, particularly pregnant women, those who are overweight, and those who must stand up a lot in their work, some of the valves give way. This allows blood to flow back down and widen the vein. However, pain and malfunction are always associated with tension, and this is at the root of the symptoms. This needs more research, but I think it is a "running away" syndrome, a resistance to being in a particular condition or situation that produces chronic tension and the resulting swelling, fatigue, pain, and valve failure. Theoretically, a resolution of the conflict ought to allow the body to repair the veins, but I don't know whether this has ever been done.

The Ankles

Our feelings of self-sufficiency, of our ability to support ourselves, are frequently reflected in the condition of our ankles. Though the knees play a role, this is where the main support of our body is focused when we are standing. If the ankles give way, we fall (or fail). So considerable tension can be located here, producing swollen or thickened ankles and various types of injuries. A sprained ankle, or even a broken one, may additionally be the body's solution to getting out of an undesirable situation, or possibly a punishment for acting against one's conscience.

The Feet

There are so many feelings and beliefs reflected here that it is hard to do justice to all of them.

Conflicts about "standing on your own two feet" may generate problems here. Flat feet or fallen arches may represent a subconscious desire to feel more "grounded" and secure about one's position or status, which word, as you probably know, is based on the verb "to stand".

Chronically curled down toes may be an attempt to get a more secure footing in life, while curled up ones might be an attempt to rise above or get away from something. Crossed over toes might be crowding together as a kind of fear reaction.

There is a system of healing called "foot reflexology" or "zone therapy," which is based on the concept that there are "reflex points" on the soles of the feet that correspond to other areas and organs of the body. When other parts of the body are out of order, these points are supposed to respond with a more or less sharp pain under applied pressure. Physiologically, such a correspondence seems impossible, and only one of the points — right in the center — is related to the acupuncture system. Nevertheless, from personal experience I can state that massaging these points definitely affects the rest of the body. It doesn't seem to make sense, but it works. So a thorough foot massage with kneading pressure, and even a good soak to relax the feet, can make you feel better all over. Maybe the sole of the foot is the "soul" of the body. Who knows?

With this chapter we end the discussion of body regions. Incomplete though it may be, its main purpose has been to get you thinking in terms of the body as a mirror of your thoughts and feelings. The next few chapters will show you how you can change those reflections you prefer not to have.

Part III — Techniques

Chapter Twelve

Idea Therapy

The emphasis of the techniques given in this chapter is on working directly with your ideas about yourself and about your life as they relate to your health. There will naturally be some overlapping with the other therapies to be given, but don't be bothered by fine distinctions. My categories are pretty arbitrary and are designed to give you a basic framework for study and practice. In actuality, you will probably end up combining techniques from several therapies, and that's as it should be.

Conflict Resolution

By now you are aware that illness is based on some internal conflict of ideas. Once that conflict is resolved, the body begins to heal itself. The most direct way to resolution is to face the ideas themselves and give one of them up. This is most easy when one of the ideas is in the "should" category. For instance, if you get a headache because you think you should do something better or differently than you are doing it, give up that idea. Sometimes you can do this by simply saying to yourself, "Why should I?" And if you get an upset stomach because someone else is not doing what you think they should do, then say, "Why should they?" and accept the fact that they don't. The use of this technique is applicable to any idea conflicts, but it does require that you be aware of what they are. To bring these to light, other techniques may be needed. Does it sound like this is easier said than done? Of course it is. It all depends on how badly you want to get well.

Re-interpretation

One of the ways in which we make our own reality is in how we interpret events. If someone criticizes you, you can interpret that as a sign of your own incompetence or as an attack which you have to defend against, or you can just as easily interpret it as a sign of the other person's lack of insight. How you interpret it can definitely affect your health.

My son once came down with flu symptoms after losing a watch. He interpreted the event as a severe loss which he was helpless to do anything about, producing an irreconcilable tension. By getting him to see that there was no trouble in getting another watch and that even if that one were lost there would be thousands of others available, he was able to reinterpret the event as a loss about which he *could* do something, and his symptoms were gone in an hour.

In another case, I worked with a woman writer who interpreted a "rejection" from a magazine as a rejection of herself, and several symptoms resulted. Simply by getting her to interpret the event as the magazine choosing not to use the article, rather than calling it a "rejection," the symptoms were relieved. Words have tremendous power because they can trigger so many emotional associations. When you know that a particular event is at the root of your physical symptoms, examine carefully the words you are using to describe the event to yourself and see whether there are other valid ways of describing it that will change the emotional effect.

Determined Intent

This is an act of will, and an extremely powerful healing technique. All it takes is a full commitment to get well, a determined intent to do so.

Every time you direct your intent toward some objective, all the resources of your mind, body, and spirit begin to flow along that path, and you start to attract events, circumstances, and people which can help. So many people, however, inhibit that flow by doubts and fears, confuse it by having conflicting or ever-changing intents, or sidetrack it by such futile ideas as "Maybe I'm supposed to be sick."

Doctors have frequently stated that one of the most, if not *the* most, important factors in cases of serious illness is the patient's will to live, his determined intent to get well no matter what. I'm telling you that the same thing is true even if we're talking about a cold or athlete's foot. Virtual miracles can occur when the will is applied in this fashion. It takes no strain or struggle, just the unwavering intent to get well. Not desire, mind you, but *intent.* Not "I want to get well," or "I really hope I'll get well," but "I'm *going* to get well."

Forgiveness

Surprised to see forgiveness listed as a technique? Don't be. Forgiveness involves a rearrangement of ideas that takes a fair amount of skill for it to be effective. An amazing number of people don't know what it really means or how to do it.

One major difficulty arises because of a confusion between forgiving and remembering. Apparently the phrase "forgive and forget" has become so ingrained in our culture that the two words are interchanged with potentially disastrous results. Often, when I've recommended that a person forgive someone who hurt them, he or she will say "You expect me to forget what they did to me?" I have to explain that I don't want them to forget, but to forgive. *Forgiveness has nothing at all to do with forgetting!* It could be silly, stupid, or even dangerous to actually forget what someone did to hurt us because then it would be impossible to learn from the incident and either avoid it or prevent it in the future. What most people do who think they are forgiving, however, is to suppress all the emotional pain (which is always on the verge of awareness and which can cause physical pain) and to try to avoid thinking about the matter (which seldom works).

The word "forgive" comes from Old English, and its root meaning is "to give away" or "to release." As we use it, it really means to release the idea that the person who hurt us should be punished. Or, in other words, to give up the idea of revenge, either by ourselves, by other people, by fate or by a righteous God. When the desire for revenge is given up, then the chronic tension that is usually associated with it is also released, resulting in more rapid healing. Sometimes, of course, we need to forgive ourselves more than anyone else. Guilt (the feeling that we should be punished), causes just as much, if not more, illness as resentment (the feeling that others should be punished). When the idea of punishment is released, so is the emotional pressure, the muscular tension, and the associated illness.

A second major difficulty people have with forgiveness is that they think all it takes is saying "Okay, I forgive." But forgiveness is not a statement, it is an act, a real act of giving up a habitual way of thinking. There is a sure-fire way to test yourself to see whether you have truly forgiven yourself or another. When you can recall, in detail, an incident that used to bring up feelings of guilt or resentment without experiencing those feelings, then forgiveness has taken place.

Now, how do you go about practicing the technique of forgiveness? There are two ways — a direct method and an indirect one.

The direct method consists of changing the belief that you or someone else deserves to be punished. While this can be incorporated into the last technique in this chapter, it can also be applied by firmly stating "I deserve (or he/she deserves) to be released from that" *every time* that a guilt or resentment feeling or memory pops into your mind. And then you direct an idea/feeling of love or blessing to the person involved. You do this in spite of what you believe at present, because you are attempting to change that belief and achieve release. A student of mine once said, "But I can't send any love to that person at this point." I explained that it didn't have to be a whole lot of love right away, just enough to start the process. After some haggling, she finally agreed that she would at least be able to send a half-inch ball of love for one second without any trouble. I told her that was fine, since she hadn't sent any at all before, and that she was to increase the amount as soon as she comfortably could. After a couple months she was up to sending a six-foot ball (in the form of pink light) for a full minute, and she was achieving the benefits of a full release.

The indirect method is simplicity itself, and has several ways of being applied. It consists of carrying out a punishment severe enough to satisfy the belief that punishment should occur. When that level of punishment has been reached, forgiveness (the release of the idea that punishment is due) is automatic. Unfortunately, when carried out on a physical level against others it leads to feuds, vendettas, individual killings and maimings, and a wide variety of emotional vengeance. And that almost always gives unsatisfactory results. When carried out against oneself, it may lead to physical injury, disability and long-term severe illness, which is also quite unsatisfactory. Some people have gotten around this by a kind of substitute punishment called "penance." This can range from wearing a hair shirt or self-maiming to saying a few prayers or fasting. Penance only works, though, when the person involved believes the punishment has been sufficient to expiate the guilt.

A much better use of the indirect method is through imagination. Since it is your subconscious or Active Mind which harbors the habitual belief in the need for punishment, and since it can't tell the difference between a "real" and a potent "imaginary" experience, then a properly imagined punishment may just provide the necessary release. The good thing about this is that it can be applied to others as well as yourself. What you do is to have a rousing daydream, in full color, and using all your senses, in which the person against whom you feel resentment is punished just as severely as you believe they deserve. The same applies if you want to get rid of guilt. After the experience, you tell yourself "Well, that's over. They (I) have been punished enough and can now be forgiven." And if some lingering resentment or guilt appears at a later date over the same incident, recall the punishment scene and remind yourself that payment has already been meted out.

The main objection to the above method that I have heard comes from people who are afraid that such thoughts might harm the other person, (this is where they believe the other deserves punishment, but they wouldn't dream of carrying it out themselves), or possibly bring similar things upon themselves. I have to tell them that, in the first place, they aren't so god-like that they can harm someone with a few thoughts. Thankfully, everyone is spiritually protected from what others actually think, or this planet would rapidly become depopulated. In the second place, it is repetitive, concentrated thought that influences our physical experience, not a single imagined incident. One intensive imagined punishment session ought to be enough. I don't recommend you go through it every day. You just need to convince your Active Mind that the experience was "real" enough to be effective, i.e., that the punishment was enough to merit forgiveness. When used with common sense, this method is harmless and very beneficial.

To give you an example of how this can work out, a man came to me with a physical problem related to guilt over some relatively minor thefts he had committed when younger. He expressed an interest in the indirect method of forgiveness, and so we went through a highly detailed daydream in which he was brought to trial. A list of his offenses was read off by an official (for some reason it was a nineteenth century court), and he was condemned to a punishment of thirty lashes. He was tied to a pole, his back was bared, and the lashes were counted off, one by one. The daydream was so intense that the man actually winced each time the imaginary whip landed. When the punishment was over, the official posted a notice on the pole to the effect that "This man has received all the punishment he deserves for these crimes, He is therefore completely forgiven and is free to go." Afterward, the man reported a tremendous sense of relief and a surge of confidence that he was now truly free of guilt that had hounded him for years. The last I heard he was fully recovered.

Inspirational Reading

When you read something interesting, you automatically go into an altered state of consciousness that resembles meditation. In this state your Active Mind is also more amenable to suggestion, as evidenced by the emotions you may feel while reading a particularly moving passage. Because of this, reading can be used as a way of incorporating healthy new beliefs into your system.

For this to be really effective, however, you have to go about it in the right way. One reading of a book, for example, no matter how moving it may be, is generally not enough to alter a habitual belief system if the ideas in the book are much different than your ordinary way of thinking. To get the greatest effect, you want to select books that contain inspirational ideas which you would *like* to believe, and then inundate your body-mind with these ideas by many and frequent readings of a series of similar books. I won't be so brash as to choose your books for you, but I would recommend those which emphasize self-knowledge, your own innate healing abilities, and those which give you a sense of spiritual uplifting.

The effectiveness of your reading, in terms of beneficial changes in your beliefs, will be enhanced by doing a relaxation exercise like the one in Chapter Three just before you start to read.

Direct Belief Changing

The most direct way to incorporate (in the sense of getting your body-mind to accept it and act accordingly), a new belief is to form it into a single, simple sentence or statement and program it into your system.

The more basic the belief, the more far-reaching effects it will have, so you want to choose a new one with care and be certain you want to live with it. For instance, if you are always or frequently sick, you might want to choose a belief like "I am always healthy." Be aware, however, that this will mean giving up all the possible side benefits you might have experienced from being ill, like getting sick leave from work or school or getting people to wait on you and sympathize with you. Or you might want to start out with something a little less basic and easier to build up your confidence in the process, like "I am immune to colds (or flu, or poison ivy)." That's what I did, with excellent results, and only later did I tackle the more basic one. In general, you'll want to choose a belief that appears to contradict an apparent fact of life. The prerequisite to a belief change of this kind, though, is a belief that you *can* change your experience by changing your beliefs. The process goes like this:

1. Get yourself physically relaxed and comfortable.
2. Remind yourself that all facts of life are no more than opinions about reality, and that you can change your opinions and change your reality beginning now.
3. Pretend to forget everything you ever believed about the subject you're going to deal with.
4. Start repeating the new statement of belief over and over for not less than five, nor more than ten, minutes.
5. If necessary, keep your mind on the subject by using your imagination to picture the effects of the new belief.
6. Use enthusiastic emotion to give power to the programming.
7. End the session and go on about your normal routine.

You need to do this once a day, at least, and to keep doing it even after you start to witness a change in your experience until the new belief becomes another "fact of life."

CHAPTER THIRTEEN

Visual Therapy

The techniques given in this chapter rely mainly on the tool of imagination, used for symptom relief, as a means of discovering the source of health problems, or for indirectly changing attitudes and beliefs.

Direct Image Substitution

If you have practiced the exercises well from Chapter Two, or if your imagination is already well-developed, then this technique should be fairly easy. It also makes use of the Reproduction Effect from the chapter on Concentration. Basically, all it consists of is building a picture of yourself, or a particular part of yourself, as well and healthy. However, there are several ways of doing this.

The most simple way is to imagine health right where there is presently sickness. For instance, suppose you have an injured thumb or an internal organ that needs healing. All you do is imagine the part *is already* healed, and keep concentrating on that image in spite of what the present condition is. The idea is that this image will serve as a guide to the body consciousness and help it to bring about the healed condition more rapidly. Unfortunately, many people have trouble with this because the contrast is too great between the image and the existing condition.

Another way which is often more effective, is to use what I call the "See & Be" technique. This utilizes both picture and mime imagination. Here you picture in your mind's eye what the body condition would be like if perfectly healed, next you construct a 3-D image of the part (external, internal, or even the whole body) in the space in front of you, then you move that image *into* your body to "coexist" with the part that needs healing. Keep repeating this process for five or ten minutes with as much desire as you can muster for the body to take the image and start rebuilding the cells according to the healed pattern. Do this at least once a day until the condition is healed, regardless of whatever other methods you use to treat it.

A third way, which works quite well for external conditions, is to focus your attention on a part of your body that is healthy and then quickly transfer that attention to the unhealthy part while giving your body the suggestion to use the healthy part as a model for healing. As you focus on the healthy part, generate feelings of pleasure, success, and thankfulness that it is so healthy, and try to maintain these feelings as you transfer your attention to the other part. This will probably be easier to apply when opposite body parts are involved. It may be advisable to cover the unhealthy part with something so that when you transfer your attention to it you can more easily imagine it as being just as healthy as the other part. I've had great success with this technique in dealing with cold sores. What I do is look in the mirror and cover up the sore with my hand so I can focus on the healthy side of my lip. And of course the results are best when this is done at the first indication that an unhealthy condition is forming. Since cold sores are often reactions to repressed retorts against criticism, I also relieve the tension by verbally blasting whoever is involved, in my imagination or out loud, when I'm alone. Never feel obliged to stick with one technique at a time if they can be conveniently used together.

Symbolic Action

This very creative technique uses the natural inclination of the Active Mind to react to extremely literal symbology. What you do is to get an imaginary picture of what the condition feels like, and then you use that image as a basis for altering the condition. I've helped people achieve some amazing results with this technique. A few examples will make it more clear.

In a work situation a woman complained that her chest was hurting like there was pressure on it. I asked her to give me an image of what kind of pressure it felt like. She said it was like boxes of books were piled on her chest. I said, "Okay, now imagine that several husky friends are coming over and they take the boxes off. Now, how does it feel?" With great surprise she said the pressure was gone, and that she had never experienced such quick relief before. In this case her image was especially convenient because we were then able to imaginatively open the boxes and look at the books, which gave her clues as to what started the pressure in the first place.

Another woman had a severe rash on her buttocks that appeared from time to time after certain particular emotional situations. Since it was there when she saw me I asked her for an image of what it felt like, but she was only aware of the unsightly bumps (which I never got to see, by the way). I happened to know that sculpting was her hobby, so I suggested she imagine her body as a clay model and that she was smoothing out the bumps. In minutes the rash was gone. We then began some work on her beliefs about confidence and security and today the rash is a thing of the past.

My wife came home from work quite fatigued one night, so I suggested that she imagine a bright ball of energy right above her head with a heavy electric cord coming out of it. Then I had her imaging plugging the cord into a socket in her right temple. She felt "recharged" in less than a minute.

The above cases give the impression that results can be obtained in a very short time, and most of the time that's true. But sometimes the imaginative action has to be repeated for a longer period until relief is obtained. Once I had a sharp pain that felt like a knife was stuck in my arm. So I pulled it out. However, since the relief was not immediate I had to keep pulling it out for quite awhile until the pain was completely gone. I would pull it out, and if the pain was still there I would imagine the knife in again and pull it out once more. On another occasion (years ago) I foolishly came down with the "flu," but I was bouncing with health in two days because I spent the time in bed visualizing a team of doctors from the future with a healing machine pointed at my chest sending health rays into me. That was the last time I ever had the flu.

As you can see from this, you can use the pain or the condition to suggest an image to work with, or you can create one that fits the situation.

Another type of symbolic action is to imagine yourself or others in miniature form entering your body and performing whatever reconstruction or repair work that is necessary. Some time ago there was a movie — I think it was "Fantastic Voyage" — in which a team of doctors in a submarine was supposedly actually miniaturized to the point where they could enter a patient's bloodstream and sail to a place where they could remove a bloodclot with lasers. Something similar would make excellent material for your own symbolic healing work. Keep in mind, though, that the object is to reduce tension and heal. I recall a TV program in which a psychiatrist was trying to heal herself of a deadly illness by a combination of medicine and imagery. In her image, she visualized a cell as a beleagured body of troops under attack by encircling Indians, representing the disease. Then she visualized the medicine as the cavalry coming to the rescue and destroying the Indians. Sad to say, the project was not successful. Aside from the fact that this was a TV story, I would suggest that the very nature of the imagery was working against a healing. In a real-life situation, based on the above imagery, I would have recommended that the medicine be visualized as a superb peacemaker who stopped the fighting by persuasion and established such harmony between the Indians and the troops that they could leave each other on friendly terms. The whole concept of fighting against disease often begets more tension and more problems.

Dream Change

This is a rather specialized type of symbolic therapy which can result in the healing of ideas that are behind illness. It is mostly for use with dreams of intense, unresolved conflict that may occur during an illness of any kind. This includes possible nightmares. Such dreams are likely to be symbolic representations of mental and emotional conflicts.

The technique consists of, first of all, remembering the dream, and then consciously replaying it as a daydream while making whatever changes seem appropriate in order to have it turn into a successful and satisfying experience. A great advantage of this technique is that you need have no conscious knowledge of what the dream symbols represent (though often this will become apparent anyway). It is enough that your Active Mind knows what they mean. By replaying the dream on better terms you are, in effect, acknowledging the current state of your beliefs and emotions and instituting necessary changes. If the beliefs involved are strongly ingrained, however, this may not be as easy as it sounds.

For example, I'll describe the case of a girl who had a nightmarish dream in which she was bound hand and foot and tossed into the back of a long black limousine as two muscular men dressed in black drove off with her. In the dream she felt very frightened and helpless. I suggested that she imagine herself breaking the bonds, clunking the heads of the two men together and tossing them out, and then getting in the front seat and driving the car herself. Obviously, such a replay would have beneficial effects on her feelings of competence, security, and self-worth. But it took her three months before she was able to carry out that imagery! This is because even our imagination is limited by our beliefs. My suggestion opened up new possibilities for her, but she had to exert considerable effort to realize those possibilities. You may not have as much difficulty as she did (which is rather unusual), but don't hesitate to use effort to stretch your mind.

The Inner Garden

Somewhat similar to Dream Changing, this technique differs only in that it uses consciously induced imagery which is then acted upon. In this case the theme is a garden of any type you desire. Usually, the person doing this would simply desire to imagine a garden representing his or her state of mind and then let the Active Mind produce one spontaneously. Or you could consciously construct one to your liking. In any event, there will be spontaneous elements to work with. Things to look for in your garden (which should have a water supply) that may need changing are the condition of the soil, the clarity of the water, the presence of many weeds or brambles or inappropriate vegetation, the state of any buildings or structures like fences and walls, the attitude of people or animals that may be there or wander in, and the weather. By "fixing up" your inner garden you can symbolically work out mental and emotional tensions relating to health and other situations in your life. And every once in a while you can check out your garden as a means of monitoring your subconscious reactions to events and circumstances.

The Double Circle

Very simple but often highly effective, this technique is designed to make clear the mental or emotional source of a particular health (or other) problem. In your imagination, you construct a circle and place within it an image of the existing condition that you are inquiring about, such as a sore throat, an ulcer, etc. Then you construct another circle to the left of the first one and say to yourself, "Show me the source of this condition." Within that circle will appear an image of some kind, or perhaps words, that will directly relate to the illness. It is up to your conscious self, however, to make the connection between what is presented and the condition. If it seems totally unrelated it is only because you are not willing to see the connection. Sometimes what appears could be symbolic and you might miss the meaning. In that case you simply say "Show me in another way" and let something different appear. The information can then be used as a basis for other techniques if necessary.

The Descending Sun

This is one variation of many similar techniques for focusing healing energy throughout or to a particular part of your body. You start out by imagining the sun as an extremely powerful ball of dynamic energy, getting a good sense of the brilliant light and heat that emanates from it and endowing it with super healing qualities. Then you either miniaturize it or bring a portion of it to rest in a ball about a foot in diameter right above your head. Very slowly then, keeping a sense of its power and healing nature, you bring it down through the top of your head and into your body, either allowing it to heal your whole body or concentrating it on a particular part. You can do this from five to twenty minutes, depending on your ability to concentrate. Then you imagine the part as being healed, give thanks, and let the light go back to the sun until you need it again.

Color Imagery

Your mind, body, and emotions respond to physical colors in definite though subtle ways, but they will respond even more quickly to imagined colors. I suspect this has a lot to do with the intent behind such use. At any rate, color imagination is a very handy and effective healing technique.

A lot has been written on the healing effects of various colors, and not all writers agree on what they are. I'm going to give you the results of a year of testing on 10-15 subjects, including only those effects on which there was no disagreement.

Red: Highly energizing and stimulating, sometimes to the point of inducing sexual feelings.

Pink: Energizing in a much gentler way, relaxing and expansive.

Orange: Very energizing, especially on the muscles, with a tendency to induce physical activity.

Yellow: Generally expansive, inducing feelings of joy and cheerfulness.

Gold: Generally rejuvenating and quite energizing.

Green: Generally calming and expansive.

Blue: Very calming with a strong tendency toward contracting or focusing.

Violet: More subtly calming and "difficult to describe."

For all around healing purposes, we found that pink, gold, and blue were the easiest to use. Pink seems to work best with fear-related tension, in cases of fatigue, and for stimulating repair work and hormone activity. Blue seems to work best with anger-related tension, for infections, and for reducing swelling and fever. Gold is an all-purpose color, useful when in doubt as to whether pink or blue would be better.

How do you use them? One effective way is through something called "color breathing." For this you imagine yourself surrounded by a cloud of the desired color, and then you breathe deeply, imagining the color filling your lungs and flowing through the rest of your body or to a particular spot. One night my wife and I were working late on a project and were getting too sleepy to continue. So I had both of us start "breathing pink." In a few minutes we were both wide awake and were able to finish the work. Much later, we were both lying in bed wondering why we couldn't get to sleep. Suddenly I remembered what we had done, so I suggested we both begin "breathing blue." We each fell asleep in the middle of it.

A very easy method is to visualize the color of your choice as a glowing light directly on or penetrating the area you are healing. The light can take any shape you give it, such as a ball, a beam, or a soft cloud. For internal work, it is sometimes easier to imagine the light outside of your body first, and then have it enter where it's needed.

Healing Angels

I like the idea of angels, but some prefer to call the images formed by this technique "healing guides, health advisors, or imaginary doctors." In any case, the process is one of spontaneously or consciously creating an imaginary person who acts as a personification of your own inner healing abilities and knowledge. It is a way of making intuitive information and skill available that otherwise might be blocked-out by conscious limitations.

Again, there are many ways to set this up. I will give you two easy methods, one using picture imagination and the other using mime imagination.

With picture imagination, just visualize a comfortable room, like an office, library, study or den, and furnish it any way you like. Put a button someplace labeled "Health Advisor" or any other title you prefer. Push the button, have the door open, and see who comes in. It could be anybody —someone you know or someone you've never seen before —but you can count on the fact that he or she knows exactly what's wrong with you and what to do about it. All you have to do is start asking questions about your condition and listen to the answers, which you may want to write down physically. It's possible that whoever walks through the door may not be suitable for some reason or other. In that case you can "release them from duty" and push the button again for another try. If, as rarely happens, no one comes in, then you will have to consciously construct an image based on your ideal of what such a person should be like. You can also have an imaginary treatment table set up in the room and allow the healer to work on you right there, which will be very beneficial in a very physical way.

It's about the same procedure with mime imagination, except that here you visualize the healer in your real environment sitting down to talk with you in a real chair and perhaps giving you a healing as if someone were really there. All of this is much more than just an exercise in imagination, as you will find if you develop proficiency in this technique. The knowledge given can be of tremendous benefit in practical terms, and the healings will have actual physical effects. The more vividly you can imagine these experiences, the more effective they will be. Somewhere in the back of your mind, though, remember that these are your creations, with the knowledge and healings brought about through cooperation with your own Active and Creative Minds.

CHAPTER FOURTEEN

Verbal Therapy

Verbal therapy emphasizes the effects of words on the mind, body, and emotions. It is almost always used in conjunction with other therapies (even when the therapist isn't aware of it), but there are a number of techniques in which verbal therapy is the primary tool.

One of mankind's oldest realizations is that words have power. At least it appears so. It became apparent very early that the mere expression of certain words seems to cause changes in feeling, thinking, behavior, health, and events. In many cases, this was attributed to a mysterious "magical" quality of the words themselves. So traditions grew up about special secret words and phrases that could grant great power to the user, if only he could find out what they were. And people experimented, sought, taught, and claimed exclusive knowledge of a wide assortment of charms, spells, chants, mantrams, and "words of power."

A lot of this may seem like nonsense, and a lot of it is. Nevertheless, dramatic effects are often achieved because behind the nonsense are a couple of very important truths. The first one is that words are not only symbols for ideas, they can also be symbols for intent. And as you remember from Chapter Twelve, determined intent is a powerful force. It is possible to have intent without words, but words serve to reinforce and focus intent, making its effects even stronger. And you know that some words or combinations of words seem to produce strong emotional effects because they stimulate associations of strongly emotional ideas. It isn't really the words themselves that have power — for they are merely symbols — but it's the ideas they symbolize.

A second truth is that sound is energy, and certain combinations of sounds, even in the form of words, can have definite beneficial effects on our emotional and physical systems. With this brief background, then, let's get on to a discussion of techniques.

Direct Command

Ever been criticized for talking to yourself? Then learn to laugh at your critic. It's a time-honored practice among those who feel a need to prepare themselves mentally, physically and emotionally for some upcoming endeavor. In this case it's called "psyching yourself up," and it's used by athletes, executives, lecturers and politicians to stimulate and focus their energy. I've heard that John F. Kennedy used to repeat "Go! Go! Go!" to himself in order to keep up the terrific pace he set for his work, and many a person has said "Calm yourself" when they've felt themselves on the brink of losing their temper. It's done because it works, and the reason it works is that the body-mind often responds dramatically to forceful commands.

I want to make it clear that I'm distinguishing between self-command and self-suggestion (to be discussed in the next section). Direct self-command is an order, not a suggestion or a statement. The latter certainly have their place, but the process is different.

In direct command you give orders to yourself that you expect to be carried out. Specifically, you give the orders to your subconscious, to your body, or to parts of your body. For instance, you might say, "Calm yourself down!" or "Relax those muscles!" or "Heal yourself!" or "Reduce that pressure!" or "Get rid of that infection!" or anything else appropriate. You can talk to yourself as a whole or you can talk to a toe, a stomach or a particular muscle. Don't be concerned with philosophical speculations as to whether or not your toe really understands what you say. Attention focuses your energy and your intent is translated by your Active Mind into whatever your toe can understand.

Like I said, results can be dramatic, but I suspect that this technique works better for those who have been trained to obey orders at some time in their life and who have a reasonable amount of self-esteem. It may not work as well for those who rebel against all authority, nor for those whose self-esteem is so low that they don't believe themselves worth listening to, even by themselves.

Auto-Suggestion

Auto- or self-suggestion is a more gentle approach than direct command. It consists of repeating suggestions, statements, or affirmations to yourself over and over until your body-mind begins to act accordingly. It's really just the reversal of a common process that may take place in your daily life when you or others suggest yourself into illness . As an example, if you frequently describe yourself as sick, weak, tired, or susceptible to illness, those words act as self-suggestions which either bring on illness or hinder your natural healing. On the other hand, listening to the unhealthy suggestions of others *without internal contradiction* can be just as bad if not worse. Pardon me if you've heard this one, but there is a story of some kids in a high school psychology class who decided to experiment on a friend. The first person who saw the friend, a girl, in the morning told her she didn't look too well, although the girl said she felt fine. The second person came up and asked if she were sick or something and she said she didn't think so. By the time several more did the same thing the poor girl accepted their suggestions, got sick, and had to go home. In such a case, mental "cancelling" of the suggestions and reaffirming a state of health and well-being would have overcome the effect. Normally, you won't receive such an intensive attack of negative suggestion, but there is enough of it around to make healthy self-suggestion a worthwhile technique to remember.

The suggestions themselves can be in line with what was discussed in the chapter on affirmation, recalling from the above section that the suggestions can be directed to specific body parts as well as to your whole self.

Rhymes and Song Substitution

Poetry was considered so special by the ancient Greeks that they put a goddess in charge of it. One reason was that they found that poetry could reach the soul (subconscious) more directly and more quickly than prose or ordinary speech. For some mysterious reason it could generate profound emotional effects and was also easier to remember. In quite a few cultures those in charge of healing found that very good results were obtained when the healing suggestions were phrased in the form of rhyming chants. Sometimes the chants would be directed to gods and spirits, but they would still be absorbed and remembered by the sick person's subconscious.

There is no need for you to seek out a particular healing chant from some far-off land, because it isn't so much the words as the rhyming cadence itself which works. All you have to do is make up your own rhyme of a healing nature, and you will end up with a form of self-suggestion that has a tendency to reach deep into your subconscious and stick. Here are a couple samples to stimulate your own creativity:

> The power of life
> Is flowing in me;
> My body is healing
> Perfectly.

and:

> With strong intent
> And powerful feeling,
> My body receives
> A perfect healing.

Of course, you can put any other part or condition in place of the word "body."

Not only do rhymes tend to stick with us, but so do certain tunes or melodies. Some companies spend a great deal of money developing jingles that are catchy, and then they simply add the words that promote their particular brand of soft drink, chicken, or whatever. Some of the tunes are so well designed to reach the subconscious that very small children learn them more quickly than what they are taught at school. What I'm recommending is that you take advantage of this by substituting your own healing affirmations for the jingle lyrics and let them start conditioning you in a healthy way. In this case, you don't have to make it rhyme because the tune itself provides the rhythm. A simple phrase like "I am healing now" can be adapted to any tune that has a tendency to catch in your mind. The repetition of the single phrase accompanied by the catchy melody can be very effective.

There's one more way to use this which differs only slightly from the above. Here you take advantage of your subconscious receptivity to any music that you hear. What you do is substitute your healing phrase for the words to any song that you may be listening to on a radio, record player, tape, etc. A great time to practice this is while driving or sitting in a car, waiting in a line or an office, or any time you have music for your ears and time on your hands.

The Five-Minute Focus

This resembles the belief-changing technique described in Chapter Twelve, with the difference that in this one you are clearly using the Reproduction Effect of concentration by programming for changes in your physical condition. You compose a statement that represents the condition you desire, worded as if it were already a fact. You repeat it over and over for five minutes, reinforcing it, if necessary, with images of the new condition and with positive feelings of enjoying the new condition. Again, you start the session by reminding yourself that you make your own reality and pretending that nothing else exists except the present unformed moment. Although you may be tempted to combine the belief changing session with this one, keep them separate for better results.

Sounding

Some people would call this chanting, but I prefer to reserve that term for the repetition of words or phrases whose primary purpose is to program information into the subconscious. "Sounding" is the term I use for the repetitive expression of sounds that may or may not be in the form of recognizable words or phrases and which may or may not have any meaning, but which do produce a therapeutic effect.

Many people are now familiar with such sounds in the form of "mantrams," usually associated with Hindu or Yogic practices, though the concept is used in quite a few other philosophical and religious systems. Generally, the purpose of monotonously repeating the mantram or sound is to gain a particular meditative state or altered state of consciousness, and it can work quite well for this. Some medical studies have shown that this practice can relieve stress and produce certain health benefits by inducing a generalized state of physical relaxation. From experience, I am convinced that the right sounds will also stimulate your biological energy flow, which can produce even more healing benefits.

There is considerable controversy over which sounds produce the best effects. Dr. Herbert Benson, who has carried out some of the studies mentioned above, feels that the word is of relatively little importance, and has achieved very good results by simply repeating "One" in conjunction with deep breathing and sitting quietly for ten to twenty minutes. But the results might just as easily be obtained from the deep breathing and sitting quietly. In fact, this could be said even for some of the religious and semi-religious systems which combine sounding with deep breathing and physical stillness. The metaphysical philosopher, J. Krishnamurti, has said that the word "Coca-cola" will do as well as any other word in such a setting. Practiced this way it becomes simply a way of obtaining the

Altered State Effect of concentration as described in Chapter Four.

Now, there is nothing wrong with that, and it can be very healthy, but what I'm about to suggest is a little different. Through a lot of experimentation I've found that certain sounds, including some traditional ones used for meditation, can produce therapeutic effects on their own without special breathing and without sitting still for so long. They can be used while driving, walking, just waiting around, or even while performing uninteresting tasks. It is my opinion that much of the benefit comes from the physical vibration that these sounds generate, which induces muscular relaxation through micro-massage and also stimulates your flow of bioenergy. I could be wrong about *how* it works, but that doesn't matter as much as the fact that for many people it *does* seem to work.

In my experience, one of the best sounds for this purpose can be spelled "AUM," though actually it is a combination of several sounds. Written out as it would sound in practice, it is like "aaaaa-ooooo-mmmmmmm," with the "m" sound being carried out longer than the others. It's best if the sound is drawn out, but there's no set length for it. To get the benefits, all you do is repeat the sound three or more times. Naturally, the more you repeat it the more you give it a chance to work, but I haven't found any particular increase in benefit after about five minutes. It can be done silently, but I think the effects are greater if done aloud, even softly. You may be able to experience clearly the bioenergy flow effect by sitting comfortably with your hands, palms up, on your lap. Pay attention to how your hands feel, then sound the above word three or four times and pay attention to your hands again. You might feel an increase in sensation, like a tingle. As an alternative, hold your palm a couple of inches above any flat surface and sound the word. The sensation may be even more pronounced. That demonstrates that your energy is flowing, and that's good for you.

Chapter Fifteen

Emotivational Therapy

Emotivational therapy is most directly involved in freeing and stimulating the flow of energy in your body. Or, if you prefer, you could say that it is the most directly involved in releasing tension. Nonetheless, it is primarily for symptom relief. I don't mean to imply that there is anything wrong with symptom relief. Sometimes it is absolutely necessary to relieve symptoms so we can get clear-headed enough to deal with the ideas that caused them. And sometimes when we relieve the symptoms of an illness the cure takes care of itself. However, you must be aware that sometimes it doesn't because relieving a symptom is an entirely different matter than bringing about a cure, and this is just as true for Imagineering as it is for orthodox medicine. If the idea behind the illness doesn't change (automatically or not), then symptom relief will only be temporary.

Still, relieving the pain of an illness is a good way to start, and although this is the last type of therapy being discussed in this book it is usually the first one I teach to my students. The main reason for that is that it happens to be the easiest to teach and to use. I believe that the widespread application of emotivational therapy alone would generate dramatic consequences that would totally change the practice of American medicine.

Therapeutic Touch

In Chapter Three I talked about bioenergy fields and currents and now I'm going to tell you how to put that information to very practical use.

Probably the oldest of humanity's healing agents is bioenergy, usually transferred from one person to another. It is often associated in people's minds with charismatic religious groups (where the technique is called "laying on hands"), with esoteric practices such as Yoga, or with specially gifted "psychics." However, the fact of the matter is that everyone (including you!) has the latent ability to use this natural energy for healing purposes without any extended or complicated training. Like anything else, the more you do it the better you get at it. But the process is so easy to learn that your greatest difficulty will be accepting that fact. I know it's easy because I first learned how to do it on my own and I have taught a great many others how do do it within a few minutes.

Fortunately, the development of this inherent healing ability is gaining both in popularity and respectability. As one example, it is part of the Master's program in nursing at New York University and is being taught to more and more nurses around the country. Someday it may even get into the doctors' curriculum, which would be a great step forward. Still, it's important to realize that it works just as well without a professional background.

As far as I know, the term "therapeutic touch" was first used by Dr. Dolores Krieger, a professor of nursing at NYU. It is an excellent term because it makes the process sound less mysterious, which is a good thing. But it is slightly misleading because often the best effects are achieved with the hands held a few inches above the skin, rather than actually touching. Why this is so, is a matter of some debate.

Attempts to explain what is happening range from simple suggestion (by the most skeptical), to electron transfer resonance (by the most scientific). As for myself, I use the working theory (which means that it works, even though it may not turn out to be exactly right) which says it involves a conscious focusing and intensification of our natural bioenergy field and current. The process is carried out by means of directed thought and emotion. Some people, of course, are unconsciously doing this very thing. They are the ones around whom you automatically feel more peaceful, energetic, or whatever. The conscious process can be even more effective, though. And just as you may not know how your muscles operate in order for you to walk, so you do not have to know exactly how therapeutic touch works in order to use it.

Since this is primarily a book of self-healing, I am not going to explain here all the ways in which you can use this technique to help others. Instead, I am going to describe how you can use it on yourself, which is a possibility overlooked by many therapeutic touchers.

If you have the idea that this technique involves a high-energy person giving energy to a low-energy person, then you may well wonder how it's possible to use it on yourself when you are in a supposedly ill or low-energy state. If that were true, then of course it wouldn't make sense. But according to my working theory, illness is brought on by localized tension which blocks or inhibits energy flow, not by a lack of energy. I believe that when a therapeutic toucher does his or her thing the effect is to promote an increase of current flow and a release of tension. Then the body is able to take over with its own natural healing processes that were inhibited by the blockage. Regardless of the explanation, the fact is that you can use it on yourself, and that is borne out by many experiences.

Your handiest tools for therapeutic touch are your hands, specifically your palms and fingertips. Normally, these are areas where your bioenergy field is very intense, and you can increase this intensity in a very simple way. During my studies of Hawaiian and African healers, I found that they would frequently rub their palms quite briskly before applying them to a patient. Trying this myself I discovered that, beside the tingling effect, there was an odd and slight sense of pressure experienced when I held my palms facing about six inches to a foot apart. Further experiments showed that I could increase that sense of pressure by imagining and desiring "more" energy coming out of my hands. When I applied my hands to others by holding them a few inches above the skin, they reported sensations of tingling, warmth, or current flow, and gradually I experienced the same sensations when I held my hands above my own skin. Even more impressive, I found that by doing this I could relieve many of my own symptoms, whether they were on the surface of my skin or inside my body. Based on what I did and have taught others to do, then, here are some suggested steps for self-applied therapeutic touch:

1. Take two or three deep breaths and relax your muscles, or use one of the relaxation exercises already described. This isn't absolutely necessary, but it helps a lot.

2. Rub your palms briskly for fifteen to thirty seconds.

3. Hold your palms six inches to a foot apart and imagine that there is an energy field between them getting stronger and stronger. This should only take a few seconds. At this point don't be concerned as to whether you feel it or not. That will come by itself.

4. Place your hands just above the area to be treated and imagine that the energy is entering the area and healing the condition. It may be helpful to imagine the energy as having a particular color. If the condition is inside the body, just imagine the energy penetrating to do its work. Personally, I like to hold my hands slightly cupped and angled inward as if the energy were being focused toward the spot, but do what feels best for you. Add any affirmations that feel appropriate. If it seems that the energy is waning, rub your hands again and reapply. You can do this for as long as you want, but I rarely do it for more than five minutes at a time, and usually less. Yes, imagination plays an important role; yes, suggestion is also a factor; and yes, there is actually an energy effect.

5. If the part of your body that you want to treat is out of reach, get as near to it as you comfortably can and imagine that the energy is flowing to it, which it will do.

Tracing

Somewhat akin to therapeutic touch, this technique is often used as part of a practice called applied kinesiology which a growing number of chiropractors are employing. Tracing involves moving the hand or fingers along certain invisible lines on the body identified as "meridians" in Chinese acupuncture. My innovation (as far as I know), is to apply the technique to yourself. Since all explanations of how this works are theoretical, I'll dispense with them except to suggest that the tracing action probably stimulates your bioenergy current flow.

Since this is a self-applied endeavor, we'll deal with only three tracing lines or meridians. One can be imagined as a line extending from the center of your chest over to the underside of your left arm, down the arm and out to the tip of your little finger. The second line extends from the same point along your right arm. The third line runs right up the center of your body.

To carry out the tracing you can use your palm or your fingertips. To trace the left side, you start with your right hand at the center of your chest and move it along the line to your left little finger in a smooth sweeping motion, repeating this at least three times. Tracing the right side is similar, except that you use your left hand, of course. The central line can be traced with either hand by moving it from your groin upward past your forehead. By moving the hands in these directions you will tend to produce a tonifying or strengthening effect which can relieve pain and tension associated with fear, depression, and fatigue. Tracing in the *opposite* direction will tend to produce a calming effect when that is desirable. No special preparation is necessary, though you may find that relaxing and rubbing your hands first will give you better results.

Plunging Into Pain

One of the worst symptoms of illness is pain, so you might think I'm crazy to suggest increasing your awareness of it. Pain is something to get rid of, not encourage, right?

Well, yes; but, nevertheless, one of the most curious effects I've run across is that paying more attention to pain often does get rid of it. In some manner that I still don't understand the increased awareness seems to relieve the tension that produces the pain.

For instance, in the case of a sudden pain from a bump or a blow against a stationary object it seems like the most natural thing to do is to move away from the object and clutch the part that hurts and hold it still while you attempt to shut the pain off. However, if this ever happens to you again, try repeating the movement that caused the contact immediately afterward for about a half dozen times, without actually touching the object. Most of the time the pain will very rapidly diminish or disappear. I know it goes against your natural inclinations, but try it anyway.

With other kinds of pain, instead of trying to pull away from it, plunge right into it and really be aware of it. Let yourself feel it completely as a pure experience without judging, criticizing, or complaining. Often it will diminish or disappear in five or ten minutes. As an alternative you may be able to analyze it out of existence. This process involves asking yourself questions about the pain and answering them no matter how odd or irrelevant they seem. The following questions can serve as a guideline. In every case, you should come up with some kind of an answer:

What shape is it? (round, square, oblong, etc.)
How big is it? (length, width, depth, in inches or feet)
How much does it weigh?
What color is it?
How fast does it move? (in miles per hour or cycles per second)
How old is it?
How much is it worth (in dollars and cents)

By the time you finish your complete analysis it may be gone, or at least reduced considerably.

Induced Arousal

This is a spin-off from the emotional inducement technique in Chapter Three. There I stated that both anger and compassion can be very arousing and healthy emotions. Not only can they shake off depression and lethargy, but they can, in certain circumstance, actually get rid of symptoms of illness and play an important role in bringing about a cure. Compassion is a form of love, and my wife, who works as a consultant for convalescent hospitals, told me of an elderly lady who was so bedridden with aches and pains that she couldn't even get dressed to go and eat in the cafeteria. That is, until an attractive and ambulatory male patient was admitted who seemed to take a liking to her. In a short time she was dressing herself and having meals with him in the dining room, and most of her symptoms were gone or greatly improved.

But it seems as if compassion or love is more easily stimulated from outside, and if that circumstance doesn't make itself available, then anger is another valid approach. I'm not advocating anger directed at any person or thing, but a profound and arousing anger at the limitations of illness itself. It is this kind of anger that has made athletes out of cripples, and it can make a healthy, vigorous person out of you, no matter what your condition. Because when you get angry enough at limitations you can break through them, and you'll be throwing aside the ideas that gave rise to them in the first place. Of course it may not be easy, because the suppression of anger may be part of your problem , but if you don't figure out some way to get your emotions flowing you may just keep sinking. Emotions are the most powerful, and therefore the most potentially healthy, form of energy there is.

CHAPTER SIXTEEN

COOPERATIVE HEALING

The primary emphasis of this book has been on self-healing, on what you can do on your own to improve your health. Such an emphasis is needed to counteract the widespread mechanical approach that fosters an almost complete dependence on someone or something else to do the healing for you. In this society, doctors, psychiatrists, psychologists, psychic and faith healers, hypnotists, and others are given god-like or demi-god status in terms of what they are expected to accomplish for a person's health. At the same time, medicines, herbs, diets, exercises and massages are endowed with magical qualities for the same end. As long as this kind of situation lasts, the healing process will remain highly expensive and only partially effective. Until you realize that *you are the only true source of your healing,* you are likely to continue to give more power to people and things than they deserve and more than they even have. It should be understood that the title of "healer" is one of courtesy rather than fact. It would be more accurate to call such a person a "healing helper."

We Need Helpers

The practice of self-healing doesn't require that you turn down help or refuse to seek it out. In a lot of cases that is simply dumb. Yet I find myself frequently having to remind my students of that. The tendency is strong in all of us to go to extremes in discarding old ideas and embracing new ones. When one realizes how dependent one has been on others for one's own health, there's a temptation to say, "Very well, from now on I won't depend on anybody!'

If you think about it for a bit you'll see that there is no such thing as complete independence, in health or in anything else. We are dependent on the earth and its living creatures for air, food, and water; and we are dependent on other people for goods, services, knowledge, and emotional fulfillment. In neither case, though, is it a one-way dependency. Instead, there is a great interdependence, a great and necessary cooperation that takes place consciously or unconsciously, willingly or unwillingly. How well it works is a matter of how well we make it work.

With healing in particular, we often need help in the form of people who have useful knowledge, skills, techniques, energy, and/or love, and it often happens that we can make practical use of supplemental factors like medicine, diets, vitamins, exercise, etc. Using any of these is not a sign of weakness; rather, it is a sign of intelligence when done with an understanding that these people and things are for helping you to heal yourself, not for making you healthy. It will help to remember these main ideas:

> **The Whole Point of Healing is to Get Healthy — Not to Prove a Method. Use What Works for You.**

In the following sections I'll give you some ideas on how to practice cooperative healing.

How To Cooperate With Food, Medicine, Exercise, Etc.

There's no need for a long exposition on this. Using the mental tools you've already learned in this book, simply affirm to your body what effects you desire from whatever is involved, and imagine the results taking place. I can't tell you what to take or do, nor when to take it or do it. For this, you have to listen to the advice of experts and then do what feels right for you. The more comfortable you feel with it, and the more convinced you are of its effectiveness, the better it will work for you. I would only recommend that you not undertake something as a result of automatic obedience to an "authority" or out of fear of what might happen if you don't undertake it. Decide whether the medicine, the exercise, or whatever, is going to help you heal yourself, and then, if you decide it will, use it with that purpose in mind.

How To Cooperate With Doctors

The following comments apply to the medical profession in general, and of course they do not take into account the particular backgrounds and ideas of individual doctors.

First of all, when I speak of "cooperating" with a doctor, I'm not referring to the kind of blind obedience and unquestioning agreement that is too often meant by that term. What I mean is the dictionary definition of "acting or working together," which means that what you do is just as important (actually more, since it's your body), as what the doctor does. You are the healer, the doctor is the helper. Now I'll briefly discuss two kinds of doctors you're likely to deal with — body doctors (including medical doctors, surgeons, chiropractors, homeopaths, acupuncturists, etc.) and mind doctors (psychiatrists, psychologists, hypnotherapists, etc.).

Body doctors are highly skilled, intensively trained, master mechanics. They know a great deal about how the body functions as a mechanism, although there are a great many new things even about that aspect of it that they don't know. Much of their information about illness is based on theory because much of their training involved the study of dead, not living, people. As a rule, they are not trained in the mental and emotional aspects of illness and are either uncomfortable in that area or hostile to it. They also have a tendency to emphasize one particular method of treatment (the one they spent so much time, effort, and money to be trained in) as *the* best method, and to be very uneasy about the value of other methods. Nevertheless, there are times when their skills can be extremely useful. Whenever I think I need the services of a master body mechanic I don't hesitate to call on one. At the same time, I realize that I am hiring them to help me, and that however skilled they may be the best they can do is to foster my own healing process. Where your body is concerned, you are the boss and the body doctor is the hired expert. Hear him out, question whatever you don't understand or don't agree with, and "co-operate" with any treatment program by using his methods to supplement your own imagineering work.

Mind doctors are also usually highly skilled and intensively trained, but they are dealing with something far less tangible than a physical body, namely ideas and emotions. Generally they are very good at labelling symptoms, but they tend to forget that a label is not an explanation. Most mind doctors follow a particular "school" of thought (Freudian, Jungian, Behaviorist, etc.) which emphasizes certain techniques over others, and they tend to give the credit to any relief or cures to the technique rather than the person. The fact is that no one has ever been cured by a technique, just as no one has ever been cured by a drug. Techniques and drugs can be useful in helping the body to heal itself, but they don't work by themselves. A good mind doctor is a master of self-awareness techniques and usually has a great fund of generalized knowledge about the mind and emotions, and about their interaction with the body. Their knowledge is much more generalized than that of a body doctor because two human bodies, which can be directly observed, have much more in common than two human minds, which cannot be directly observed. Taking into account their own personal beliefs and prejudices, mind doctors often have sound advice to give on effective ways of thinking and relating. So they can be hired to teach you self-awareness techniques and to give you advice on better ways of channeling your thoughts and emotions. But since a mind doctor cannot know *your* mind or *your* emotions, you get the best use out of one by choosing from what they have to say the techniques and advice that you feel will best help you. Be open enough to try anything you don't feel is absolutely wrong, but keep only what works for you.

How To Cooperate With Psychic Healers

You may or may not ever use one, but nevertheless there are quite a few good psychic healers around. By "good" I mean those who are honestly trying to help people and who are quite effective at what they do. What they do, by and large, is to share with you an abundant supply of bioenergy to aid your body's healing process, along with giving you healing-oriented suggestions. The only way I know of to determine whether a psychic healer is "good," is either to ask others who have gone to him (her) or try one out and see how you react. Like doctors, a psychic healer may be caught up in believing that his method or technique can cure you, but don't let that stop you from making use of the extra energy he may be able to supply you. Such a healer is also no more than a hired expert whom you can use to supplement your own healing. The better your rapport with the healer, the better the results you will get. If you are skeptical, consider trying one anyway — you may be surprised. If you are fearful, I recommend that you skip this form of aid unless you get over the fear, because that will interfere with any possible benefit. If you should decide to try a psychic healer — as a supplement to your personal healing efforts — be sure to realize that you are free to combine or add this type of treatment to whatever you are receiving from doctors. They are not mutually exclusive, at least not in terms of treatment. Sometimes the doctors and the psychic healers themselves don't get along too well, but that's their problem, not yours. Remember, your aim is to get healed so don't hesitate to draw from whatever resources are available while remembering that you are the prime healer.

How To Cooperate With a Friend

Imagineering is a personal process, but it is a lot easier to do when that process is shared and aided by a friend. That friend could be a relative, a frequent companion, or an acquaintance, as long as you both agree on the validity of what you are doing. You can help each other by doing the various exercises together, perhaps taking turns to guide each other through them, by reminding each other of the available techniques and meanings of the body regions, and by sharing bioenergy whenever one or the other needs it. Imagineering is more fun and more effective when you can do it with someone else.

How To Start A Healing Cooperative

By far the best way to practice Imagineering is to get together with a group of peole who want to learn how to heal themselves and who are willing to help others do it, too. By combining your ideas, your energies, resources, reinforcement, and encouragement, you can bring about substantial and even dramatic improvements in the health of the whole group. I know this for a fact because this has been the experience of the co-ops that I have already formed. The oldest of these has been in operation for about seven years and its membership has ranged from three to about twenty-five. Now, I'm not going to tell you that everyone in the co-op is always in perfect health, but a number of them are who never used to be and most of the rest are healthy far more of the time than they are ill. When they do fall ill for reasons personal to them, they are quickly supported and aided back to health by the other members. Within the group, colds, flu, and other minor ailments are extremely rare and don't last long when they do appear. Most co-op members visit doctors a lot less because they need them a lot less, and some have forgotten what a doctor's office looks like. Those who have had accidents recovered faster than expected and those few with serious illness (originating before joining the group), receive all the support they can handle.

There is no set way to form such a healing cooperative, so I will merely make some suggestions based on my experience. The main thing is the desire to help each other become and stay healthier.

Organization

1. Keep it simple. All you really need is a leader or organizer who will be responsible for setting up and guiding meetings and activities. You don't have to bother with officers and committees. Stay informal, make any decisions by group consensus, and work toward building such a spirit of mutual support that there will always be volunteers for anything that has to be done. In this kind of atmosphere (one could call it a loving one), cooperative healing can flow freely.
2. Have regular weekly meetings, if you can. This acts like a "recharge" to keep people thinking in terms of health and self-healing. If you can't meet weekly, meet twice a month. Meet once a month if you can't do anything else, but your group will cease to be effective if you meet less often than that.
3. Three to seven people is a very good size for a healing cooperative. If the group gets much larger than that then a strong leader and some reorganization is necessary. One solution is to have the larger group divided into smaller ones, with the large group meeting once a month and the smaller ones weekly. Another solution is to have the large group meet weekly and the smaller groups either meet monthly or more often at different times. The larger the group, the more it tends to turn into a passive audience with a few active leaders. This may be helpful as a way of imparting knowledge, but it is no longer a cooperative. Keep the actual co-ops small, and if a lot of people get interested then you can have general meetings of different co-ops that also have their own meetings.
4. If your group starts to get larger than seven people, *and* if you happen to have someone with a bit of literary talent, you might want to put out a simple

one- or two-page newsletter containing healing ideas and techniques, reviews of healing books, and inspirational quotes.

5. As long as your group is quite small you shouldn't have to be concerned with dues or such, but if it gets to the point where costs of refreshments, a newsletter, and such things may be burdensome, then have your group decide on something reasonable to cover expenses.

Activities At Meetings: (choose your own order)

1. Study Time. This is for the discussion and demonstration of ideas and techniques on self-healing, and for the relating of personal experiences with healing. An easy way to do this is to have someone read a passage from a book on self-healing (either the present one or some other one of interest), and then discuss what was read and try out any techniques that may have been mentioned.

2. Healing Time. This is the time to work directly with the members present. Group meditation is one way, guided by someone who gives healing suggestions to everyone present. Or the group may want to listen to a meditation or healing tape, of which there are many on the market. A very effective practice is to have a person who needs healing sit in the center of the group while the others direct healing energy to him or her with their hands, as described in Chapter Fifteen, and give silent or whispered healing suggestions. If desired, each person can take a turn sitting in the center. The individual being helped will, of course, be doing his or her own inner work at the same time.

3. Social Time. To build a good group rapport there definitely should be some social time just for gabbing and sharing refreshments. Sometimes a surprising amount of healing can take place at this time in a spontaneous way. I do recommend, however, that the social time come at the end of the meeting if you want to get anything else done.

Non-Meeting Activities:

1. Healing Hot Line. I think that this is one of the most important activities of the co-op. What it means is that any co-op member can feel free to call another when they need healing help, reinforcement, encouragement, or information. It is very strengthening to know you have someone to call on in time of need. If the person who is called doesn't feel capable of helping alone, then that person calls the other members of the co-op either to call the one who needs help or to set up an emergency meeting. Most of the time, however, the one in need just needs a voice of encouragement or an idea or two.

While writing the last chapter, I received a call from a co-op member whose daughter had just developed a high fever as they were preparing to go on vacation. She said she was thinking of taking the girl to the doctor that afternoon. I told her that was a good idea, but in the meantime, I asked if anything had happened to upset the girl. It turned out that the girl had just had a bad argument with her brother. So I suggested that the mother have the girl "beat up" her brother in her mind and call me back later. The mother knew about this idea but had forgotten it in the concern of the moment. Not long after, the mother called to say the girl's temperature was back to normal and that she had gotten a real kick out of the exercise.

Well, this brings me to the end of the book. I've shared with you a bundle of ideas, theories, experiences, and techniques in the hope that at least some of you will find something that will help you to become healthier and happier. Much as I might like to, I can't do a single thing *for* you, and neither can anyone else. But the purpose of this book is well expressed in these lines from Lord Byron:

> Words are things, and a small drop of ink
> Falling like dew upon a thought, produces
> That which makes thousands, perhaps millions, think.

More "self-help" books published by Quest

Art of Inner Listening — *By Jessie Crum*
"So you would like to be a genius," writes the author. Simply stop talking — and listen — really listen.

The Choicemaker — *By E.B. Howes & S. Moon*
Man and his intrinsic need to make choices.

Concentration — *By Ernest Wood*
Will help you take full charge of your mind.

Do You See What I See? — *By Jae Jah Noh*
How to live fully, indeed passionately, with no inner conflicts.

Mastering the Problems of Living — *By Haridas Chaudhuri*
Overcome depression! Conquer anxiety! Make decisions!

The Path of Healing — *By H.K. Challoner*
Based on the holistic nature of all life. Heal yourself with harmonious living.

A Way to Self-Discovery — *By I.K. Taimni*
A way of life book for serious students of the "ancient wisdom."

Available from:
The Theosophical Publishing House
306 West Geneva Road, Wheaton, Illinois 60187